GERIATRICS *At Your* FINGERTIPS™

2004, 6th EDITION

AUTHORS:

David B. Reuben, MD

Keela A. Herr, PhD, RN, FAAN

James T. Pacala, MD, MS

Bruce G. Pollock, MD, PhD

Jane F. Potter, MD

Todd P. Semla, MS, PharmD

PUBLISHED BY BLACKWELL PUBLISHING, INC.
MALDEN, MA, USA

This publication was prepared by Blackwell Publishing, Inc., at the direction of the American Geriatrics Society as a service to health care providers involved in the care of older persons.

Although *Geriatrics At Your Fingertips* ™ is distributed by various companies in the health care field, it is independently prepared and published. All decisions regarding its content are solely the responsibility of the authors. Their decisions are not subject to any form of approval by other interests or organizations.

Some recommendations in this publication suggest the use of agents for purposes or in dosages other than those recommended in product labeling. Such recommendations are based on reports in peer-reviewed publications and are not based on or influenced by any material or advice from pharmaceutical or health care product manufacturers.

No responsibility is assumed by the authors or the American Geriatrics Society for any injury or damage to persons or property, as a matter of product liability, negligence, warranty, or otherwise, arising out of the use or application of any methods, products, instructions, or ideas contained herein. No guarantee, endorsement, or warranty of any kind, express or implied (including specifically no warrant of merchantability or of fitness for a particular purpose) is given by the Society in connection with any information contained herein. Independent verification of any diagnosis, treatment, or drug use or dosage should be obtained. No test or procedure should be performed unless, in the judgment of an independent, qualified physician, it is justified in the light of the risk involved.

Citation: Reuben DB, Herr KA, Pacala JT, *et al. Geriatrics At Your Fingertips: 2004, 6th Edition.*
Malden, MA: Blackwell Publishing, Inc., for the American Geriatrics Society; 2004.

ISBN 1-4051-0443-0
Library of Congress Catalog Card Number 2003022516
Printed in the U.S.A.

GERIATRICS *At Your* FINGERTIPS™

2004, 6th EDITION

TABLE OF CONTENTS

AUTHORS

David B. Reuben, MD
Director, Multicampus Program in Geriatric Medicine and Gerontology
Chief, Division of Geriatrics
Professor of Medicine
David Geffen School of Medicine at UCLA
Los Angeles, CA

Keela A. Herr, PhD, RN, FAAN
Professor
Chair, Adult and Gerontological Nursing
College of Nursing
The University of Iowa
Iowa City, IA

James T. Pacala, MD, MS
Associate Professor and Vice Chair for Medical Student Affairs
Distinguished Teaching Professor
Department of Family Practice and Community Health
University of Minnesota School of Medicine
Minneapolis, MN

Bruce G. Pollock, MD, PhD
Professor of Psychiatry, Pharmacology, and Pharmaceutical Sciences
Chief, Academic Division of Geriatrics and Neuropsychiatry
Department of Psychiatry, University of Pittsburgh
Pittsburgh, PA

Jane F. Potter, MD
Chief, Section of Geriatrics and Gerontology
Harris Professor of Geriatric Medicine
University of Nebraska Medical Center
Omaha, NE

Todd P. Semla, MS, PharmD
Associate Professor
The Feinberg School of Medicine
Northwestern University
Chicago, IL

ABBREVIATIONS

ABG	arterial blood gas
ACC	American College of Cardiology
ACE	angiotensin-converting enzyme
ACIP	Advisory Committee on Immunization Practices
ACOG	American College of Obstetrics and Gynecology
ACR	American College of Rheumatology
AD	Alzheimer's disease
ADA	American Diabetes Association
ADLs	activities of daily living
AFB	acid-fast bacillus
AGS	American Geriatrics Society
AHA	American Heart Association
AHRQ	Agency for Healthcare Research and Quality (formerly, Agency for Health Care Policy and Research)
AIDS	acquired immune deficiency syndrome
AIMS	Abnormal Involuntary Movement Scale
ALT	alanine aminotransferase
APAP	acetaminophen
ASA	acetylsalicylic acid or aspirin
ASA class	American Society of Anesthesiologists grading scale for surgical patients
ATA	American Thyroid Association
ATS	American Thoracic Society
AUA	American Urological Association
BIPAP	bilevel positive airway pressure
BMD	bone mineral density
BMI	body mass index
BP	blood pressure
BPH	benign prostatic hyperplasia
BUN	blood urea nitrogen
C&S	culture and sensitivity
CABG	coronary artery bypass graft
CAD	coronary artery disease
CBC	complete blood cell count
cfu	colony-forming unit
CHD	coronary heart disease
CI	confidence interval
CMS	Centers for Medicare and Medicaid Services (formerly, US Health Care Financing Administration, or HCFA)
CNS	central nervous system
COPD	chronic obstructive pulmonary disease
CPAP	continuous positive airway pressure
CPK	creatine phosphokinase
CPR	cardiopulmonary resuscitation
Cr	creatinine

CrCl	creatinine clearance
CT	computed tomography
CXR	chest x-ray
CYP	cytochrome P-450
D&C	dilation and curettage
D5W	dextrose 5% in water
DBP	diastolic blood pressure
D/C	discontinue
DHIC	detrusor hyperactivity with impaired contractility
DSM-IV	*Diagnostic and Statistical Manual of Mental Disorders*, 4th ed. (Washington, DC: American Psychiatric Association; 1994)
DVT	deep-vein thrombosis
ECF	extracellular fluid
ECG	electrocardiogram, electrocardiography
EF	ejection fraction
EPS	extrapyramidal symptoms
ESR	erythrocyte sedimentation rate
FDA	Food and Drug Administration
FEV_1	forced expiratory volume in 1 second
FOBT	fecal occult blood test
FVC	forced vital capacity
GAD	generalized anxiety disorder
GDS	Geriatric Depression Scale
GERD	gastroesophageal reflux disease
GFR	glomerular filtration rate
GI	gastrointestinal
GU	genitourinary
Hb	hemoglobin
HbA_{1c}	glycosylated hemoglobin
HCFA	*See* CMS
HCTZ	hydrochlorothiazide
HDL	high-density lipoprotein
HF	heart failure
HR	heart rate
HT	hormone therapy
HTN	hypertension
hx	history
IADLs	instrumental activities of daily living
IBW	ideal body weight
INH	isoniazid
INR	international normalized ratio
IOP	intraocular pressure
IPC	intermittent pneumatic compression
JNC 7	Seventh Joint National Committee on Prevention, Detection, Evaluation, and Treatment of High Blood Pressure
K^+	potassium ion
LBW	lean body weight
LDL	low-density lipoprotein

LDUH	low-dose unfractionated heparin
LFT	liver function test
LMWH	low-molecular-weight heparin
LVH	left ventricular hypertrophy
MAOI	monoamine oxidase inhibitor
MI	myocardial infarction
MMSE	Folstein's Mini–Mental State Examination
MSE	mental status examination
MRI	magnetic resonance imaging
NG	nasogastric
NSAIDs	nonsteroidal anti-inflammatory drugs
NPH	neutral protamine Hagedorn (insulin)
OCD	obsessive-compulsive disorder
OGTT	oral glucose tolerance test
OT	occupational therapy
PE	pulmonary embolism
PEF	peak expiratory flow
PET	positron emission tomography
PNS	peripheral nervous system
POMA	Performance-Oriented Mobility Assessment
PPD	purified protein derivative (of tuberculin)
PSA	prostate-specific antigen
PT	prothrombin time *or* physical therapy
PTCA	percutaneous transluminal coronary angioplasty
PTT	partial thromboplastin time
PUVA	psoralen plus ultraviolet light of A wavelength
QT_c	QT (cardiac output) corrected for heart rate
RBC	ranitidine bismuth citrate *or* red blood cells
sats	saturations
SD	standard deviation
SBP	systolic blood pressure
SIADH	syndrome of inappropriate secretion of antidiuretic hormone
SOB	shortness of breath
SPECT	single-photon emission computed tomography
SPEP	serum protein electrophoresis
SSRIs	selective serotonin-reuptake inhibitors
TCA	tricyclic antidepressant
TD	tardive dyskinesia
TDD	telephone device for the deaf
TG	triglycerides
TIA	transient ischemic attack
TSG	thyroid-stimulating globulin
TSH	thyroid-stimulating hormone
TTP	thrombotic thrombocytopenic purpura
TUIP	transurethral incision of the prostate
TURP	transurethral resection of the prostate
U	unit(s)
UA	urinalysis

UI	urinary incontinence
UV	ultraviolet
VIN	vulvar intraepithelial neoplasia
WHO	World Health Organization
wt	weight

Drug Prescribing and Elimination

Drugs are listed by generic names; trade names are in *italics*. Check marks (√) indicate drugs preferred for treating older persons. Formulations are bracketed and expressed in milligrams (mg) unless otherwise specified. Abbreviations for dosing, formulations, and route of elimination are defined below.

ac	before meals
bid	twice a day
C	capsule, caplet
conc	concentrate
CR	controlled release
crm	cream
ChT	chewable tablet
d	day(s)
ER	extended release
F	fecal elimination
gran	granules
h	hour(s)
hs	at bedtime
IM	intramuscular(ly)
Inj	injectable(s)
IT	intrathecal(ly)
IV	intravenous(ly)
K	renal elimination
L	hepatic elimination
lot	lotion
max	maximum
MDI	metered-dose inhaler
min	minute(s)
mo	month(s)
npo	nothing by mouth
NS	normal saline
oint	ointment
OTC	over-the-counter
OU	both eyes
pc	after a meal
pk	pack, packet
po	by mouth
pr	per rectum
prn	as needed

pwd	powder
qam	every morning
qd	every day
qhs	each bedtime
qid	four times a day
qod	every other day
S	liquid (includes concentrate, elixir, solution, suspension, syrup, tincture)
SC	subcutaneousl(ly)
sec	second(s)
shp	shampoo
sl	sublingual
sol	solution
Sp	suppository
spr	spray(s)
SR	sustained release
sus	suspension
syr	syrup
T	tablet
tinc	tincture
tid	three times a day
TR	timed release
wk	week(s)
yr	year(s)

INTRODUCTION

Providing high-quality medical care for older persons requires a special set of knowledge, clinical skills, and attitudes. Many resources contain current, accurate information on evaluation and management of the older patient. However, few are portable enough to be used in the examining room, on nursing home or hospital rounds, or when the clinician is on call outside the office.

In 1998, the American Geriatrics Society (AGS) first published *Geriatrics At Your Fingertips™* (*GAYF*), a pocket guide that provides immediate access to specific information needed to care for older persons in various health care settings. The response was extraordinary, and *GAYF* soon became the society's best-selling publication. During the past two years, the AGS has created new platforms for *GAYF* to take advantage of the expanding integration of electronic mediums into clinical practice. Specifically, beginning in 2002, *GAYF* became available on the Internet (www.geriatricsatyourfingertips.org) and in 2004, *GAYF* will become available in Palm and Windows CE operating systems. Clinicians will then be able to have *GAYF* instantly available on their PDAs.

In this edition, we added a table of common herbal and alternative medications used by older adults, including side effects and cautions. New sections on syncope, skin ulcers, carpal tunnel syndrome, and hospital discharge planning have also been added. We have updated information throughout the text and tables, including recommended diagnostic tests, management strategies, and assessment instruments. Tables and lists of drugs are designed to facilitate appropriate prescribing. Generic and trade names are provided, as well as information on dosages, how the drugs are metabolized or excreted, and which formulations are available. Specific caveats and cautions to be observed when using the medication in older persons are also included.

The goal of *GAYF* is to reduce to a minimum the amount of time that a practicing clinician must spend searching for specific information that is needed immediately to make patient care decisions. Accordingly, the book does not attempt to explain in detail the rationale underlying the strategies presented. In many instances, these strategies have been derived from guidelines published by organizations such as the Agency for Healthcare Research and Quality, the American Geriatrics Society, the American Heart Association, and the American Diabetes Association. Many of the guidelines can be obtained from the National Guidelines Clearinghouse (www.guideline.gov). When no such guidelines exist, the strategies recommended herein represent the best opinions of the authors and the experts they have asked to review the chapters. In an effort to be comprehensive yet concise, references have been provided sparingly, but many others that are relevant are available from the organizations mentioned or in the most recent edition of the AGS *Geriatrics Review Syllabus*.

The authors welcome comments about the format and content of this edition of *GAYF* that may guide the preparation of future editions. All comments should be addressed to the American Geriatrics Society, Empire State Building, 350 Fifth Avenue, Suite 801, New York, NY 10118.

The authors are particularly grateful to Nancy Lundebjerg at the AGS, who has served a vital role in the development of this book and its readership. We are also grateful to the John A. Hartford Foundation for support in distributing *GAYF* to residents and medical and nurse practitioner students across the nation and for generously supporting the development of PDA versions.

We would also like to thank the following persons who have reviewed parts of this edition:

Lodovico Balducci, MD
Perry Fine, MD
Rita A. Frantz, PhD, RN
Gail Greendale, MD
Catherine MacLean, MD, PhD

Patrick E. McBride, MD, MPH
Lauren Nathan, MD
Larissa Rodriguez, MD
Paul Tuite, MD
Thomas T. Yoshikawa, MD

Guidelines of the following organizations are the basis of parts of specific chapters:

Advisory Committee on Immunization Practices
Agency for Healthcare Research and Quality
  (formerly, Agency for Health Care Policy and Research)
Alzheimer's Association
Amercian Academy of Neurology
American Association for Geriatric Psychiatry
American College of Cardiology
American College of Chest Physicians
American College of Gastroenterology
American College of Obstetrics and Gynecology
American College of Rheumatology
American Diabetes Association
American Geriatrics Society
American Heart Association
American Lung Association
American Pain Society
American Psychiatric Association
American Society of Anesthesiologists
American Thyroid Association
American Urological Association
Ethnogeriatrics Committee, American Geriatrics Society
National Cholesterol Education Program
National Heart, Lung, and Blood Institute
U.S. Preventive Services Task Force
World Health Organization

The following persons have assisted the authors in planning and assembling the 2004 edition:

Managing Editor: Carol S. Goodwin
Medical Editor: Susan E. Aiello, DVM, ELS
Medical Indexer: L. Pilar Wyman, Wyman Indexing

FORMULAS AND REFERENCE INFORMATION

Table 1. Conversions		
Temperature	**Liquid**	**Weight**
$F = (1.8)C + 32$	1 fl dram = 4 mL	1 lb = 0.453 kg
$C = (F - 32) / (1.8)$	1 fl oz = 30 mL	1 kg = 2.2 lb
	1 tsp = 5 mL	1 oz = 30 g
	1 tbsp = 15 mL	1 grain = 60 mg

FORMULAS

Alveolar-Arterial Oxygen Gradient $A - a = 148 - 1.2(Paco_2) - Pao_2$
[normal = 10 − 20 mm Hg, breathing room air at sea level]

Calculated Osmolality
2Na + glucose / 18 + BUN / 2.8 + ethanol / 4.6 + isopropanol / 6 + methanol / 3.2 + ethylene glycol / 6.2   [normal = 280 – 295]

Golden Rules of Arterial Blood Gases
• Pco_2 change of 10 corresponds to a pH change of 0.08.
• pH change of 0.15 corresponds to base excess change of 10 mEq/L.

Creatinine Clearance
For renally eliminated drugs, dosage adjustments may be necessary if CrCl < 60.

$$\frac{IBW(140 - age)\,(0.85\ \text{if female})}{(72)\,(\text{stable creatinine})}$$

Erythrocyte Sedimentation Rate
Westergren: women = (age + 10) / 2
          men = age / 2

Ideal Body Weight
• Male = 50 kg + (2.3 kg) (each inch of height > 5 feet)
• Female = 45.5 kg + (2.3 kg) (each inch of height > 5 feet)

Lean Body Weight
IBW + 0.4 (actual body weight − IBW)

Body Mass Index

$$\frac{\text{weight in kg}}{(\text{height in meters})^2} \quad or \quad \frac{\text{weight in lb}}{(\text{height in inches})^2} \times 704.5$$

Partial Pressure of Oxygen, Arterial (Pao$_2$) While Breathing Room Air
100 − (age/3) estimates decline

Table 2. Motor Function by Nerve Roots			
Level	Motor Function	Level	Motor Function
C4	Spontaneous breathing	L1–L2	Hip flexion
C5	Shoulder shrug	L3	Hip adduction
C6	Elbow flexion	L4	Hip abduction
C7	Elbow extension	L5	Great toe dorsiflexion
C8/T1	Finger flexion	S1–S2	Foot plantar flexion
T1–T12	Intercostal abdominal muscles	S2–S4	Rectal tone

Table 3. Lumbosacral Nerve Root Compression			
Root	Motor	Sensory	Reflex
L4	Quadriceps	Medial foot	Knee-jerk
L5	Dorsiflexors	Dorsum of foot	Medial hamstring
S1	Plantar flexors	Lateral foot	Ankle-jerk

Figure 1. Dermatomes

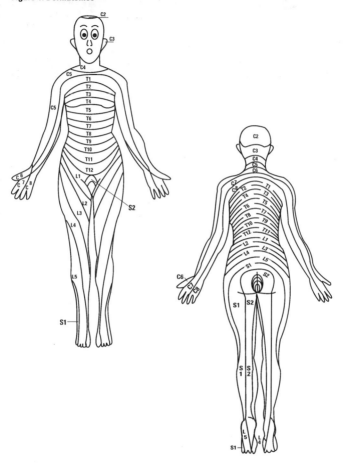

Source: *The Tarascon Pocket Pharmacopoeia*, 2003 edition. Loma Linda, CA: Tarascon Publishing, 2003:79. Reprinted with permission.

ASSESSMENT AND APPROACH

ASSESSMENT

Table 4. Assessing Older Adults*			
Assessment Domain	Screening Methods	Further Assessment (if screen is positive)	See Page(s)
Medical			
Medical illnesses	Hx, screening physical examination	Additional targeted physical examination, laboratory and imaging tests	
Medications	Medications review	Pharmacy referral	9, 195
Nutrition	Inquire about weight loss (> 10 lbs in past 6 mo), weigh patient	Dietary hx, malnutrition evaluation	92
Dentition	Oral examination	Dentistry referral	
Hearing	Hand held audioscope, Brief Hearing Loss Screener	Ear examination, audiology referral	71, 186
Vision	Inquire about vision changes, Snellen chart testing	Eye examination, ophthalmology referral	174
Pain	Inquire about pain	Pain Inventory	119
Urinary incontinence	Inquire if patient has lost urine > 5 times in past year	UI evaluation	170
Mental			
Cognitive status	3-item recall, Mini-Cog, MMSE	Mental status examination, dementia evaluation	183
Emotional status	GDS or other depression screen, inquire "Do you ever feel sad or blue?"	In-depth interview	185
Spiritual status	Spiritual hx	In-depth interview, chaplain or spiritual advisor referral	
Physical			
Functional status	ADLs, IADLs	PT/OT referral	183–185
Balance and gait	Observe patient getting up and walking, orthostatic BP and HR	POMA scale	187
Falls	Inquire about falls in past year	Falls evaluation	59
Environmental			
Social, financial status	Social hx	In-depth interview, social work referral	
Environmental hazards	Inquire about living situation, home safety checklist	Home evaluation	Table 31

* See also Assessment Instruments, pp 183–196.

HOUSING ALTERNATIVES FOR OLDER PERSONS

Depending on need for assistance and financial resources, various options are available. Specific names may differ by region, and some may be combinations of various types (see also p 133).

- **Home** with support, if necessary, including caregiver (PP or limited hours if on Medicaid), home-delivered meals (usually PP with sliding scale), homemaker (usually PP with sliding scale)
- **Senior citizen housing** typically does not provide individual services although some may have a social worker available and may provide access to hiring help (PP, may be subsidized for elders spending over one-third of income for rent)
- **Continuing care retirement communities** provide living arrangements ranging from independent to skilled (PP)
- **Assisted living facilities, residential care facilities, board-and-cares** provide meals, housekeeping services, and medication management (PP and Medicaid for some facilities)
- **Nursing homes** provide skilled and custodial care, some have separate units for dementia and behavioral problems (PP, Medicaid, Medicare only if following a 3-day or longer hospital stay)

  PP = private pay

SCHEDULED NURSING HOME VISIT CHECKLIST

1. Evaluate patient for interval functional change
2. Check vital signs, weight, laboratory tests, consultant reports since last visit
3. Review medications (correlate to active diagnoses)
4. Sign orders
5. Address nursing staff concerns
6. Write a SOAP note (subjective data, objective data, assessment, plan)
7. Revise problem list as needed
8. Update advance directives at least yearly
9. Update resident; update family member(s) as needed

INFORMED DECISION MAKING (see also **Figure 2**)

Physicians have no ethical obligation to offer care that is judged to be futile. Three elements are needed for a patient's choices to be legally, ethically valid:

- A capable decision maker: Capacity is to the decision being made; patient may be capable of making some but not all decisions. For a sufficiently impaired person, a surrogate decision maker must be involved.
- Patient's voluntary participation in the decision-making process.
- Sufficient information: Patient must be sufficiently informed; items to disclose in informed consent include:
  - Diagnosis
  - Nature, risks, costs, and benefits of possible interventions
  - Alternative treatments; relative benefits, risks, and costs
  - Likely results of no treatment
  - Likelihood of success
  - Advice or recommendation of the clinician

Figure 2. Informed Decision Making

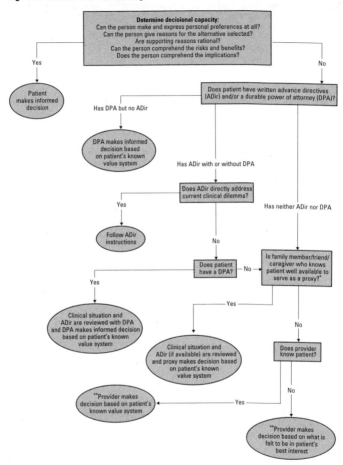

ELDER MISTREATMENT

Risk Factors for Inadequate or Abusive Caregiving

- Cognitive impairment in patient, caregiver, or both
- Dependency (financial, psychological, etc) of caregiver on elderly patient, or vice versa
- Family conflict
- Family history of abusive behavior, alcohol or drug problems, mental illness, or mental retardation
- Financial stress
- Isolation of patient or caregiver, or both
- Living arrangements inadequate for needs of the ill person
- Stressful events in the family, such as death of a loved one or loss of employment

Source: Fulmer T. Elder mistreatment. In: Cobbs EL, Duthie ED, Murphy JB, eds. *Geriatrics Review Syllabus: A Core Curriculum in Geriatric Medicine, 5th ed.* Malden, MA: Blackwell Publishing for the American Geriatrics Society; 2002:55. Reprinted with permission.

Assessment and Management

- Interview patient and caregiver separately.
- Ask patient some general screening questions, such as, "Are there any problems with family or household members that you would like to tell me about?" Follow-up a positive response with more direct questions such as those suggested in **Table 5.**
- On physical examination, look for any unusual marks, signs of injury, or conditions listed in **Table 5.**
- If mistreatment is suspected, report case to Adult Protective Services (most states have mandatory reporting laws).
- If patient is in immediate danger of harm, create and implement plan to remove patient from danger (hospital admission, court protective order, placement in safe environment, etc).

CROSS-CULTURAL GERIATRICS

Clinicians should remember that:

- Wide differences appear among the individuals in every ethnic group.
- Familiarity with a patient's background is useful only if his or her preferences are linked to the cultural heritage.
- Ethnic groups differ widely in
  - approach to decision making (eg, involvement of family and friends),
  - disclosure of medical information (eg, cancer diagnosis),
  - end-of-life care (eg, advance directives and resuscitation preferences).

In caring for patients of any ethnicity:

- Use the patient's preferred terminology for his or her cultural identity in conversation and in health records.
- Determine whether interpretation services are needed.
- Recognize that the patient may not conceive of illness in Western terms.
- Determine whether the patient is a refugee or survivor of violence or genocide.

Table 5. Signs that Raise Suspicion of Elder Mistreatment		
Type of Mistreatment	Some Clinical Signs of Possible Mistreatment	Questions to Ask Patient to Gather more Hx
Abandonment	Patient brought to clinic or emergency room by someone other than caregiver, patient dropped off and abandoned at health care facility by caregiver	Is there anyone you can call to come and take care of you?
Physical abuse	Fractures or bruises in various stages of healing, unexplained bruises, repeated falls, unexplained azotemia	Has anyone at home ever hit you or hurt you?
Exploitation	Evidence that personal belongings are being taken without consent or approval, unexplained loss of Social Security or pension checks	Has anyone taken your things?
Neglect	Dermatitis from urine in contact with skin, malnourishment, poor hygiene, inappropriate dress, listlessness or apathy	Are you receiving enough care at home?
Psychological abuse	Observed impatience, irritability, or demeaning behavior toward patient by caregiver; anxiety, fearfulness, ambivalence, or anger shown by patient toward caregiver	Has anyone ever scolded or threatened you? Has anyone made fun of you?

Source: Adapted from Fulmer T. Elder mistreatment. In: Cobbs EL, Duthie ED, Murphy JB, eds. *Geriatrics Review Syllabus: A Core Curriculum in Geriatric Medicine, 5th ed.* Malden, MA: Blackwell Publishing for the American Geriatrics Society; 2002:55-6. Reprinted with permission.

- Explore early on the patient's preferences for disclosure of serious clinical findings and reconfirm at intervals.
- Ask if the patient prefers to involve or defer to others in the decision-making process.
- Follow the patient's preferences regarding gender roles.

APPROPRIATE PRESCRIBING AND PHARMACOTHERAPY

HOW TO PRESCRIBE APPROPRIATELY

- **Obtain a complete drug history.** Ask about previous treatments and responses as well as about other prescribers. Ask about allergies, OTC drugs, nutritional supplements, alternative medications, alcohol, tobacco, caffeine, and recreational drugs.
- **Avoid prescribing before a diagnosis is made.** Consider nondrug therapy. Eliminate drugs for which no diagnosis can be identified.
- **Review medications regularly and before prescribing a new medication.** D/C medications that have not had the intended response or are no longer needed. Monitor the use of prn and OTC drugs.
- **Know the actions, adverse effects, and toxicity profiles of the medications you prescribe.** Consider how these might interact or complement existing drug therapy.
- **Start chronic drug therapy at a low dose and titrate dose on the basis of tolerability and response.** Use drug levels when available.
- **Attempt to reach a therapeutic dose before switching or adding another drug.**
- **Educate patient and/or caregiver about each medication.** Include the regimen, the therapeutic goal, the cost, and potential adverse effects or drug interactions. Provide written instructions.
- **Avoid using one drug to treat the side effects of another.**
- **Attempt to use one drug to treat two or more conditions.**
- **Use combination products cautiously.** Establish need for more than one drug. Titrate individual drugs to therapeutic doses and switch to combinations if appropriate.
- **Communicate with other prescribers.** Don't assume patients will—they assume you do!
- **Avoid using drugs from the same class or with similar actions** (eg, alprazolam and zolpidem).

See also Medication Appropriateness Assessment, p 195. For more on drugs that should be avoided in all elderly patients, see p 200.

WAYS TO REDUCE MEDICATION ERRORS

- Be knowledgeable about the medication's dose, side effects, interactions, and monitoring.
- Write legibly to avoid misreading of the drug name (*Celexa* versus *Celebrex*).
- Write out the directions, strength, route, quantity, and number of refills.
- Always precede a decimal expression of <1 with a zero (0); never use a zero after a decimal.
- Avoid abbreviations, especially easily confused ones (qd and qid).
- Do not use ambiguous directions, eg, as directed (ud) or as needed.
- Include the medication's purpose in the directions (eg, for high blood pressure).
- Write dosages for thyroid replacement therapy in μg not mg.
- Always re-read what you've written.

CRITERIA FOR DRUGS OF CHOICE FOR OLDER ADULTS
• Established efficacy
• Compatible safety and side-effect profile
• Low risk of drug or nutrient interactions
• Half-life < 24 h with no active metabolites
• Elimination does not change with age or known dose adjustments for renal or hepatic function
• Convenient dosing—single or twice daily
• Strength and dosage forms match recommended doses for older adults
• Affordable to the patient

PHARMACOLOGIC THERAPY AND AGE-ASSOCIATED CHANGES

Table 6. Age-Associated Changes in Pharmacokinetics and Pharmacodynamics			
Parameter	Age Effect	Disease, Factor Effect	Prescribing Implications
Absorption	Rate and extent are usually unaffected	Achlorhydria, concurrent medications, tube feedings	Drug-drug and drug-food interactions are more likely to alter absorption
Distribution	Increase in fat : water ratio; decreased plasma protein, particularly albumin	HF, ascites, and other conditions will increase body water	Fat-soluble drugs have a larger volume of distribution; highly protein-bound drugs will have a greater (active) free concentration
Metabolism	Decreases in liver mass and liver blood flow may decrease drug metabolism	Smoking, genotype, concurrent drug therapy, alcohol and caffeine intake may have more effect than aging	Lower doses may be therapeutic
Elimination	Primarily renal; age-related decrease in GFR	Renal impairment with acute and chronic diseases; decreased muscle mass results in less Cr production	Serum creatinine not a reliable measure of renal function; best to estimate CrCl using formula on p 1
Pharmaco-dynamics	Less predictable and often altered drug response at usual or lower concentrations	Drug-drug and drug-disease interactions may alter responses	Prolonged pain relief with opioids at lower doses; increased sedation and postural instability to benzodiazepines; altered sensitivity to β-blockers

COMPLICATING FACTORS
Drug-Food or -Nutrient Interactions
Physical Interactions: Mg^{++}, Ca^{++}, Fe^{++}, Al^{++}, or zinc can lower oral absorption of levothyroxine and some quinolone antibiotics. Tube feedings will decrease absorption of oral phenytoin and levothyroxine.

Decreased Drug Effect: Warfarin and vitamin K-containing foods (eg, green leafy vegetables, broccoli, brussels sprouts, greens, cabbage).

Decreased Oral Intake or Appetite: Drugs can alter the taste of food (dysgeusia) or decrease saliva production (xerostomia), making mastication and swallowing difficult. Drugs associated with dysgeusia include captopril and clarithromycin. Drugs that can cause xerostomia include antihistamines, antidepressants, antipsychotics, clonidine, and diuretics.

Drug-Drug Interactions

A drug's effect can be increased or decreased by another drug because of impaired absorption (eg, sucralfate and ciprofloxacin), displacement from protein-binding sites (eg, warfarin and sulfonamides), inhibition or induction of metabolic enzymes (see **Table 7**), or because two or more drugs have a similar pharmacologic effect (eg, potassium-sparing diuretics, potassium supplements, and ACE inhibitors).

Digoxin: Digoxin levels must be monitored with concomitant administration of many other drugs.

The following **increase** digoxin concentration or effect, or both:

amiodarone	hydroxychloroquine	quinine
diltiazem	ibuprofen	spironolactone
erythromycin	indomethacin	tetracycline
esmolol	nifedipine	tolbutamide
flecainide	quinidine	verapamil

The following **decrease** digoxin concentration or effect, or both:

aminosalicylic acid	colestipol	sulfasalazine
antacids	kaolin pectin	St. John's wort
antineoplastics	metoclopramide	
cholestyramine	psyllium	

Enzyme Inhibitors and Inducers: **Table 7** is a list of common drug-drug interactions via this mechanism.

Table 7. Selected CYP Isozyme Substrates, Inducers, and Inhibitors				
Substrates*		Isozyme	Inducers**	Inhibitors†
APAP Clozapine Desipramine Estradiol Imipramine	Nortriptyline Olanzapine Warfarin	CYP1A2	Carbamazepine Cigarette smoke Omeprazole Phenobarbital Phenytoin Rifampin	Amiodarone Cimetidine Diltiazem Estradiol Fluoroquinolones Fluvoxamine Isoniazid Ketoconazole
Celecoxib Fluvastatin Phenytoin Warfarin		CYP2C9	Carbamazepine Phenobarbital Phenytoin Rifampin	Amiodarone Cimetidine Fluconazole Fluvoxamine Isoniazid Omeprazole Propoxyphene Valproic acid
Codeine† Dextromethorphan Donepezil Haloperidol Metoprolol Most TCAs	Paroxetine Risperidone Timolol Tramadol‡ Venlafaxine	CYP2D6		Amiodarone Bupropion Celecoxib Cimetidine Diltiazem Fluoxetine Paroxetine Propoxyphene Quinidine Valproic acid

(continues)

Table 7. Selected CYP Isozyme Substrates, Inducers, and Inhibitors (cont.)				
Substrates*		Isozyme	Inducers**	Inhibitors†
Alprazolam	Lovastatin	CYP3A4	Carbamazepine	Amiodarone
Amiodarone	Nefazodone		Glucocorticoids	Cimetidine
Atorvastatin	Omeprazole		Griseofulvin	Clarithromycin
Buspirone	Pioglitazone		Oxcarbazepine	Cyclosporine
Carbamazepine	Quetiapine		Phenobarbital	Diltiazem
Clarithromycin	Risperidone		Phenytoin	Erythromycin
Clozapine	Sildenafil		Pioglitazone	Fluconazole
Codeine	Simvastatin		Rifabutin	Fluoxetine
Cyclosporine	Triazolam		Rifampin	Fluvoxamine
Dihydropyridine	Venlafaxine		St. John's wort	Grapefruit juice
calcium channel	Verapamil			Haloperidol
blockers	Warfarin			Isoniazid
Diltiazem	Ziprasidone			Itraconazole
Donepezil	Zolpidem			Ketoconazole
Erythromycin				Propoxyphene
Estradiol				Nefazodone
Fluoxetine				Quinidine
Haloperidol				Sertraline
Itraconazole				Verapamil
Ketoconazole				

* Substrate: a drug metabolized by the isozyme.
** Inducer: a drug that increases the capacity of the isozyme to metabolize the substrate and potentially decreases the therapeutic effect of the substrate.
† Inhibitor: a drug that prevents the isozyme from metabolizing the substrate and increases the risk for toxicity or therapeutic failure of the substrate.
‡ Analgesic effect decreased because of inhibition of substrate metabolism to its active metabolite by an inhibitor.
Note: The list of medications is not comprehensive, but represents medications often prescribed for older patients or medications involved in very serious drug interactions (eg, cyclosporine). Some interactions have in vivo or in vitro documentation, whereas others are theoretical. For more information, consult a drug-drug interaction text or Internet resource, eg, http://medicine.iupui.edu/flockhart/.

Table 8. Common Herbal and Alternative Medications Used by Older Adults				
Product	Common Uses	Side Effects	Drug Interactions	Cautions
Chondroitin	Osteoarthritis	Nausea, dyspepsia, changes in intraocular pressure		
Echinacea	Immune stimulant	Hepatotoxicity	Immuno-suppressants	Discontinue ≥ 2 wk before surgery; cross-sensitivity with chrysanthemum, ragweed, daisy, and aster allergies; renal disease; immuno-suppression

Table 8. Common Herbal and Alternative Medications Used by Older Adults (cont.)				
Product	**Common Uses**	**Side Effects**	**Drug Interactions**	**Cautions**
Feverfew	Anti-inflammatory, migraine prophylaxis	Platelet inhibition, bleeding, GI upset	NSAIDs, anti-platelet agents, anticoagulants	Discontinue 7 d before surgery, active bleeding
Garlic	Hypertension, hypercholesterolemia, platelet inhibitor	Bleeding, GI upset, hypoglycemia	NSAIDs, anti-platelet agents, anticoagulants	Discontinue 7 d before surgery
Ginger	Antiemetic, anti-inflammatory, dyspepsia	Bleeding	NSAIDs, anti-platelet agents, anticoagulants	Discontinue 7 d before surgery
Ginkgo	Alzheimer's disease, memory, intermittent claudication, macular degeneration	Bleeding, nausea, headache, GI upset, diarrhea, anxiety	MAOIs	Discontinue 36 h before surgery
Ginseng	Physical and mental performance enhancer	Hypertension, tachycardia	Anti-platelet agents, anticoagulants, NSAIDs, MAOIs	Discontinue 7 d before surgery, renal failure
Glucosamine	Osteoarthritis, rheumatoid arthritis	GI distress, anorexia, insomnia, painful and itchy skin, peripheral edema, tachycardia		Allergy to shellfish
Kava kava	Anxiety, sedative	Sedation	Anticonvulsants (increased effect)	Discontinue 24 h before surgery
SAMe (S-adeno-sylmethionine)	Depression, fibromyalgia, insomnia, osteoarthritis, rheumatoid arthritis	GI distress, insomnia, dizziness, dry mouth, headache, restlessness	Antidepressants, St. John's wort, NSAIDS, anti-platelet agents, anticoagulants	Not effective for bipolar depression, hyperhomocysteine-mia (theoretical), discontinue at least 14 d before surgery
Saw palmetto	BPH	Headache, nausea, GI distress, erectile dysfunction	Finasteride, alpha blockers	
St. John's wort	Depression, anxiety	Photosensitivity, hypomania		Wear sunscreen, avoid in fair-skinned patients, discontinue 5 d before surgery
Valerian	Anxiety, insomnia	Sedation, benzodiazepine-like withdrawal		Taper dose several weeks before surgery

ALCOHOL AND TOBACCO ABUSE

ALCOHOL ABUSE
Definition
Possible Alcohol Dependence—DSM-IV: Three or more of the following:
- Tolerance, requiring more alcohol to get "high"
- Withdrawal, or drinking to relieve, prevent withdrawal
- Drinking in larger amounts, or for a longer time than intended
- Persistent desire to drink, or unsuccessful efforts to control drinking
- Spending a lot of time obtaining, using alcohol, or recovering from effects
- Giving up important occupational, social, or recreational activities because of drinking
- Drinking despite persistent or recurrent physical or psychologic problems caused or worsened by alcohol

Possible Alcohol Abuse—DSM-IV: Recurring problems with one or more of the following:
- Drinking resulting in the failure to fulfill major obligations at work or in the home
- Drinking in situations where it is physically hazardous
- Alcohol-related legal problems
- Continued drinking despite social problems caused or worsened by alcohol

Hazardous Drinking: WHO definition—use of alcohol that places a person at risk of physical or psychologic complications. Increases risk of HTN, some cancers (eg, head and neck, esophagus, breast in women), and cirrhosis (higher in women). Possible increased risk for hip fracture and other injury.

Evaluation
Alcohol dependence or abuse is often missed in older persons because of reduced social and occupational functioning; signs more often are poor self-care, malnutrition, and medical illness.

Alcohol Misuse Screening: CAGE questionnaire has been validated in the older population.

C Have you ever felt you should **C**ut down?
A Does others' criticism of your drinking **A**nnoy you?
G Have you ever felt **G**uilty about drinking?
E Have you ever had an "**E**ye opener" to steady your nerves or get rid of a hangover? (*Positive response to any suggests problem drinking.*)

Detecting Harmful Drinking ($\geq$ *2 drinks/d for women,* $\geq$ *3 drinks/d for men is potentially harmful*): May be missed by CAGE; ask

- How many days per week?
- How many drinks on those days?
- Maximum intake on any one day?
- What type (ie, beer, wine, or liquor)?
- What is in "a drink"?

Aggravating Factors
Alcohol and Aging: Higher blood levels per amount consumed due to decreased lean body mass and total body water; concomitant medications may interact with alcohol.

Age-related Diseases: Cognitive impairment, HTN.
Medications: Many drug interactions, eg, APAP, antihypertensives, NSAIDs, sedatives, antidepressants.

Management
Alcohol Guidelines for Moderate Drinking: No more than 1 drink/d after age 65; 1 drink/d probably reduces cardiovascular and cerebrovascular risk.
Psychosocial Interventions:
• Problem drinking or alcohol misuse: Brief intervention; educate patient on effects of current drinking, point out current adverse effects.
• Alcohol dependence or abuse: Self-help groups (eg, Alcoholics Anonymous); professional (eg, psychodynamic, cognitive-behavioral, counseling, social support, family therapy, age-specific inpatient or outpatient).
• Drug therapy: Naltrexone *(Depade, REVIA, Trexan)* 25 mg × 2d, then 50 mg qd [T: 50]. Monitor liver enzymes; useful adjunct to psychosocial therapy; contraindicated in renal failure; ~10% get nausea, headache (L, K).
• Acute alcohol withdrawal: See p 39.

SMOKING CESSATION
Non-Pharmacologic Therapy
What Health Providers Should Do:
• **Ask** about tobacco use at every visit
• **Advise** all users to quit
• **Assess** willingness to quit
• **Assist** the patient with a quit plan, education, pharmacotherapy
Making the Decision to Quit:
Patients are more likely to stop smoking if they:
• Believe they could get a smoking-related disease
• Believe they can make an honest attempt at quitting
• Believe the benefits of quitting outweigh the benefits of continued smoking
• Know someone who has had health problems as a result of smoking
Setting a Quit Date and Deciding on a Plan:
• Pick a specific day within the next month, gives time to develop a plan
• Will nicotine replacement therapy be used?
• Will the patient attend a smoking cessation class?
• On quit day, get rid of all cigarettes and related items.
Managing Symptoms of Withdrawal:
• **Physical:** Pharmacotherapy (**Table 9**) helps physical symptoms.
• Who should/should not receive pharmacotherapy?
  - Nicotine replacement:
    ○ Improves quit rates in most patients
    ○ Is contraindicated with recent MI, uncontrolled high BP, arrhythmias, severe angina, gastric ulcer
    ○ May not be needed if patient smokes fewer than 10 cigarettes/day; if used, recommend lower dosages
  - Other agents (buproprion, etc):
    ○ May be used if nicotine contraindicated
    ○ Use in combination with nicotine if prior failure using nicotine alone

- **Psychological:**
  - Smoking is linked with many activities, and the link must be unlearned.
  - Avoid people and places where tempted to smoke.
  - Alter habits: 1) switch to juices or water instead of alcohol or coffee, 2) take a brisk walk instead of a coffee break, and 3) use oral substitutions such as sugarless gum or hard candy.
  - Three types of counseling and behavioral therapies are effective: 1) provide problem solving/skills training, 2) provide social support as part of treatment, and 3) provide social support outside of treatment.

Maintaining Smoking Cessation: Use the same methods that helped during withdrawal.

Source: Adapted from Global Strategy for the Diagnosis, Management, and Prevention of Chronic Obstructive Pulmonary Disease, Global Initiative for Chronic Obstructive Lung Disease (GOLD). NHLBI/WHO Workshop Report, Executive Summary. National Institutes of Health, National Heart, Lung and Blood Institute. March 2001. NIH Publication No. 2701A (for full report, see www.goldcopd.com).

Table 9. Pharmacotherapy for Tobacco Abuse			
Drug	**Dosage**	**Formulations**	**Comments (Metabolism, Excretion)**
Tobacco Abuse			
Bupropion* (*Wellbutrin SR, Zyban*)	150 mg bid × 7–12 wk	SR: 100, 150	Combined with nicotine replacement, doubles quit rate to 30% at 12 mo; contraindicated with seizure disorders (L)
Nicotine Replacement**			
Transdermal patches[†] (eg, *Habitrol, Nicoderm*)	21 mg/d × 4–8 wk 14 mg/d × 2–4 wk 7 mg/d × 2–4 wk	7, 14, 21	Apply to clean, nonhairy skin on upper torso, rotate sites; start 14 mg/d with cardiovascular disease or body wt < 100 lb or if smoking < 10 cigarettes/d (L)
(*Nicotrol*)	15 mg/d × 8 wk 10 mg/d × 4–6 wk 5 mg/d × 4–6 wk	5, 10, 15	Gradually released over 16 h (L)
(*ProStep*)	22 mg/d × 4–8 wk 11 mg/d × 4–8 wk	11, 22	Persons < 100 lb start lower dose; reduce or D/C after 4–8 wk (L)
Polacrilex gum (*Nicorette*)	9–12 pieces/d	2, 4	Chew 1 piece when urge to smoke; usual 10–12 d, maximum 30/d; 4 mg for smokers > 21 cigarettes/d (L)
Nasal spray (*Nicotrol NS*)	1 spr each nostril q 30–60 min	0.5 mg/spr	Do not exceed 5 applications/h or 40 in 24 h (L)
Inhaler[††] (*Nicotrol Inhaler*)	6–16 cartridges/d	4 mg delivered/cartridge	Maximum 16 cartridges/d with gradual reduction after 6–12 wk if needed (L)

* Bupropion is FDA approved. Nortriptyline is an effective alternative. Hughes JR, Stead LF, Lancaster T. Antidepressants for smoking cessation. *Cochrane Database Syst Rev* 2002; 1:000031.

** Best used in combination with smoking cessation program; dyspepsia is most common drug-related side effect.

[†] In patients receiving > 600 mg cimetidine, reduce to next lower patch dose.

[††] Available by prescription only.

ANTICOAGULATION

WARFARIN THERAPY
Prescribing Warfarin
- Initiate therapy by giving warfarin (*Coumadin, Carfin, Sofarin*) 2–5 mg/d as fixed dose [T: 1, 2, 2.5, 3, 4, 5, 6, 7.5, 10]; reduce dose if INR > 2.5 on day 3.
- Half-life is 31–51 h; steady state is achieved on day 5–7 of fixed dose.
- Warfarin therapy is implicated in **many** adverse drug-drug interactions.
- The following drugs **increase** INR in conjunction with warfarin:

alcohol use (binge)	ASA (> 3 g/d)	SSRIs
allopurinol	corticosteroids	tamoxifen
amiodarone	NSAIDs	vitamin E (≥ 400 IU)
antibiotics	omeprazole	
APAP (> 1.3 g/d >1 wk;	phenytoin	
monitor INR)	propoxyphene	

- The following drugs **decrease** INR in conjunction with warfarin:

alcohol use (moderate)	cholestyramine	sucralfate
barbiturates	estrogens	vitamin K
carbamazepine	rifampin	

Table 10. Indications for Anticoagulation in the Absence of Active Bleeding or Severe Bleeding Risk		
Condition	**Target INR**	**Duration of Therapy**
Hip or major knee surgery	2.0–3.0	7–10 days or until patient is ambulatory
Idiopathic venous thromboembolism (includes PE)	2.0–3.0 1.5–3.0	First 3 mo 3 mo–indefinitely
Atrial fibrillation	2.0–3.0	Indefinitely
Mitral valvular heart disease with hx of systemic embolization or left atrial diameter > 5.5 cm	2.0–3.0	Indefinitely
Cardiomyopathy with EF < 25%	2.0–3.0	Indefinitely
Mechanical aortic valve with normal left atrial size and sinus rhythm	2.0–3.0*	Indefinitely
Mechanical aortic valve with enlarged left atrium and/or atrial fibrillation	2.5–3.5*†	Indefinitely
Mechanical mitral valve	2.5–3.5*†	Indefinitely
Caged ball or caged disk valve	2.5–3.5‡	Indefinitely
Bioprosthetic heart valve	2.0–3.0	3 mo
Acute MI complicated by severe LV dysfunction, HF, previous emboli, mural thrombus on echocardiography	2.0–3.0	1–3 mo

* If additional risk factors are present or if there is systemic embolism despite anticoagulation treatment, target INR is 2.5–3.5 and ASA 80–100 mg/d should be added.
† Alternative target INR 2.0–3.0 with addition of ASA 80–100 mg/d.
‡ With addition of ASA 80–100 mg/d.

Cessation of Anticoagulation Before Surgery

• If INR is between 2.0 and 3.0, hold warfarin 4 doses before surgery; longer if INR > 3.0.
• If patient has a mechanical valve, heparin should be used after warfarin is held before surgery.

Table 11. Treatment of Warfarin Overdose		
INR	**Clinical Situation**	**Action**
≥ 3.5 and < 5.0	No significant bleeding	Omit next warfarin dose and/or lower dose
≥ 5.0 and < 9.0	No significant bleeding	Omit next 1–2 doses of warfarin and restart therapy at lower dose; alternatively, omit 1 dose and give vitamin K (VK) 1.0–2.5 mg po
≥ 9.0	No significant bleeding	D/C warfarin and give VK 3.0–5.0 mg po; give additional VK orally if INR is not substantially reduced in 24–48 h. Restart warfarin at lower dose when INR is therapeutic.
≥ 3.0 and < 20.0	Serious bleeding	D/C warfarin; give VK 1.0–10.0 mg by slow IV infusion, supplemented with fresh frozen plasma or prothrombin complex concentrate depending on urgency of situation; check INR q 6h; repeat VK q 12h as needed
Any elevation	Life-threatening bleeding	D/C warfarin; give VK 10.0 mg by slow IV infusion, supplemented with prothrombin complex concentrate; repeat this treatment as needed

Source: Data from American College of Chest Physicians Consensus Panel on Antithrombotic Therapy: Ansell J, Dalen J, Anderson D, et al. Managing oral anticoagulant therapy. In: Sixth ACCP Consensus Conference on Antithrombotic Therapy. *Chest.* 2001; 119(1 Suppl):22S–38S.

ACUTE ANTICOAGULATION

Table 12. Anticoagulants for DVT/PE Prophylaxis and Treatment			
Class, Agent	**DVT/PE Prophylaxis Dosage By Condition Type**	**DVT/PE Treatment Dosage**	**Comments**
Heparin			
Unfractionated heparin (*Hep-Lock*)	General surgery: 5000 U SC 2 h before and q 12 h after surgery	5000 U/kg IV bolus followed by 15 mg/kg/h IV*	Bleeding, anemia, thrombocytopenia, hypertransaminasemia, urticaria (L, K)

Table 12. Anticoagulants for DVT/PE Prophylaxis and Treatment (cont.)			
Class, Agent	DVT/PE Prophylaxis Dosage By Condition Type	DVT/PE Treatment Dosage	Comments
LMWH			
Enoxaparin (*Lovenox*)	THA, HFX: 30 mg SC q 12 h or 40 mg SC qd KR: 30 mg SC q 12 h; AS: 40 mg SC qd	Outpatient treatment of DVT: 1 mg/kg SC q 12 h; Inpatient treatment of DVT ± PE: 1 mg/kg SC q 12 h or 1.5 mg/kg SC qd*	Bleeding, anemia, hyperkalemia, hypertransaminasemia, thrombocytopenia, thrombocytosis, urticaria, angioedema (K)
Dalteparin (*Fragmin*)	Low risk THA: 2500–5000 U SC before surgery, 5000 U SC qd after surgery Abdominal surgery: 2500–5000 U SC before and after surgery	Also indicated for anticoagulation in acute coronary syndrome	Same (K)
Tinzaparin (*Innohep*)	NA	175 anti-Xa IU/kg SC qd*	Same (K)
Heparinoid			
Danaparoid (*Organan*)	THA, HFX, HIT: 750 anti-Xa U SC bid	NA	Same as LMWH (K)
Factor Xa Inhibitor			
Fondaparinux (*Arixtra*)	THA, HFX, KR: 2.5 mg SC qd beginning 6–8 h after surgery	NA	Contraindicated if weight < 50 kg or CrCl < 30 mL/min (K)
Direct Thrombin Inhibitor			
Argatroban	HIT: 2 μg/kg/min IV infusion	HIT: 2 μg/kg/min IV infusion	↓ dosage if hepatic impairment (L)
Thrombolytics			
Streptokinase (*Kabikinase, Streptase*)	NA	250,000 U IV over 30 min, then 100,000 U/h for 24 h†	Risk of hemorrhage ↑ with age and higher BMI; hypertension, hallucination, agitation, confusion, serum sickness (L)

Note: THA = total hip arthroplasty (hip replacement); HFX = hip fracture surgery; KR = knee replacement; HIT = heparin-induced thrombocytopenia; NA = not applicable
* Also indicated for anticoagulation in acute coronary syndrome (see **Table 14**).
† Dose in acute MI is 1.5 million U IV over 60 min.

DIAGNOSIS

Anxiety disorders are less prevalent in elderly than in younger adults. New-onset anxiety in elderly persons is often secondary to physical illness, depression, medication side effects, or withdrawal from drugs.

DSM-IV recognizes several anxiety disorders:
(*Italicized type indicates the most common anxiety disorders occurring in older persons.*)
• Acute stress disorder
• Agoraphobia without a history of panic
• *GAD*
• *Anxiety disorder due to a general medical condition*
• Obsessive-compulsive disorder (OCD)
• Panic disorder, with or without agoraphobia
• Post-traumatic stress disorder
• Social anxiety disorder
• Specific phobia
• Substance-induced anxiety disorder

DSM-IV Criteria for GAD
• Excessive anxiety and worry on more days than not for $\geq$ 6 mo, about a number of events or activities
• Difficulty controlling the worry
• Anxiety and worry associated with $\geq$ 3 of 6 symptoms:
  - restlessness or feeling keyed up or on edge
  - being easily fatigued
  - difficulty concentrating or mind going blank
  - irritability
  - muscle tension
  - sleep disturbance (difficulty falling or staying asleep, or restless unsatisfying sleep)
• Focus of anxiety and worry not confined to features of an Axis I disorder (primary psychiatric disorder); often, about routine life circumstances; may shift from one concern to another
• Anxiety, worry, or physical symptoms cause clinically significant distress or impairment in social, occupational, or other important areas of functioning
• Disturbance not due to the direct physiologic effects of a drug of abuse or a medication or to a medical condition; does not occur exclusively during a mood disorder, psychotic disorder, or a pervasive development disorder.

DSM-IV Criteria for Panic Attack
Discrete period of intense fear or discomfort with ≥ 4 of the following (also, must peak within 10 min):

- Palpitations, rapid HR
- Sweating
- Trembling or shaking
- Sensations of SOB or smothering
- Choking feeling
- Chest pain or discomfort
- Nausea or abdominal distress
- Feeling dizzy, unsteady, lightheaded, or faint
- Feelings of unreality or being detached from self
- Fear of losing control or going crazy
- Fear of dying
- Paresthesias
- Chills or hot flushes

Differential Diagnosis
- Physical conditions producing anxiety
  - Cardiovascular: Arrhythmias, angina, MI, HF
  - Endocrine: Hyperthyroidism, hypoglycemia, pheochromocytoma
  - Neurologic: Movement disorders, temporal lobe epilepsy, AD, stroke
  - Respiratory: COPD, asthma, pulmonary embolism
- Medications producing anxiety
  - Caffeine
  - Corticosteroids
  - Nicotine
  - Psychotropics: Antidepressants, antipsychotics, stimulants
  - Sympathomimetics: Pseudoephedrine, β-agonists
  - Thyroid hormones: Overreplacement
- Withdrawal states: alcohol, sedatives, hypnotics, benzodiazepines
- Depression

EVALUATION
- Past psychiatric hx
- Drug review: Prescribed, OTC, alcohol, caffeine
- Mental status evaluation
- Physical examination: Focus on signs and symptoms of anxiety (eg, tachycardia, hyperpnea, sweating, tremor)
- Laboratory tests: Consider CBC, blood glucose, TSH, B_{12}, ECG, oxygen saturation, drug and alcohol screening

MANAGEMENT
Nonpharmacologic
- Cognitive-behavior therapy may be useful for GAD, panic disorder, and OCD.
- May be effective alone but mostly used in conjunction with pharmacotherapy.
- Requires a cognitively intact, motivated patient.

Pharmacologic
Antidepressants Approved for Anxiety Disorders: See **Table 25** for dosing.
- Obsessive-compulsive: fluoxetine, fluvoxamine, paroxetine, sertraline; secondary choices include β-blockers and atypical antipsychotics
- Panic: sertraline, paroxetine; secondary choices include β-blockers and atypical antipsychotics
- Social anxiety disorder: paroxetine
- Generalized anxiety: venlafaxine, paroxetine
- Post-traumatic stress: paroxetine, sertraline

Buspirone (BuSpar):
- Serotonin 1A partial agonist effective in GAD and anxiety symptoms accompanying general medical illness
- Not effective for acute anxiety, panic, or OCD
- May take 2–4 wk for therapeutic response
- Recommended geriatric dosage: 15–20 mg bid [T: 5, 7.5, 10, 15, 30]
- No dependence, tolerance, withdrawal, CNS depression, or significant drug-drug interactions

Benzodiazepines:
- Most often used for acute anxiety, GAD, panic, OCD
- Preferred: Intermediate–half-life drugs inactivated by direct conjugation in liver and therefore less affected by aging
- Long-acting benzodiazepines (eg, flurazepam, diazepam, chlordiazepoxide): Linked to cognitive impairment, falls, sedation, psychomotor impairment
- Problems: Dependence, tolerance, withdrawal, more so with short-acting benzodiazepines; seizure risk with alprazolam withdrawal
- Potentially fatal if combined with alcohol or other CNS depressants
- Only short-term (60–90 d) use recommended

Table 13. Benzodiazepines for Anxiety Recommended for Geriatric Patients		
Drug	**Dosage**	**Formulations**
Lorazepam (*Ativan*)	0.5–2 mg in 2–3 divided doses	T: 0.5, 1, 2; S: 2 mg/mL; Inj: 2 mg/mL
Oxazepam (*Serax*)	10–15 mg bid–tid	T: 10, 15, 30

CARDIOVASCULAR DISEASES

CORONARY ARTERY DISEASE
Diagnostic Cardiac Tests
- Cardiac catheterization is the gold standard.
- Stress testing: The heart is stressed either through exercise (treadmill, stationary bicycle) or, if the patient cannot exercise or the ECG is markedly abnormal, with pharmacologic agents (dipyridamole, adenosine, dobutamine). Exercise stress tests can be performed with or without cardiac imaging, while pharmacologic stress tests always include imaging. Imaging can be accomplished by a nuclear isotope (eg, thallium) or echocardiography.
- Electron-beam computed tomography (EBCT) is not currently recommended as a screening test for CAD.

Acute Myocardial Infarction
Evaluation and Assessment
- Presentation frequently atypical—suspect MI with atypical chest pain; arm, jaw, or abdominal pain (with or without nausea); acute functional decline.
- As in younger persons, diagnosis is made by cardiac enzyme rises, with or without ECG changes. Serial enzyme measurements are necessary to exclude MI.
  - Both creatine kinase MB isoenzymes (CK-MB) and cardiac troponins T and I usually become elevated 4 h following myocardial injury.
  - CK-MB subforms are the most sensitive and specific test for detecting MI in the first 6 h, but troponin remains elevated longer.
  - Elevated troponin in the face of normal CK-MB can indicate increased risk of MI in the ensuing 6 mo.
  - Troponins are not useful for detecting reinfarction within first wk of an MI. CK-MB is the preferred marker for early reinfarction.
  - Both CK-MB and cardiac troponins can exhibit false-positive results that are due to subclinical ischemic myocardial injury or nonischemic myocardial injury.
- Risk factors for acute MI in older adults:

  Strong:
  - Previous MI or angina
  - Age
  - Diabetes mellitus
  - Hypertension
  - Smoking
  - Severe coronary artery calcification

  Weak:
  - Dyslipidemia (except in those with overt coronary disease)
  - Family hx
  - Obesity
  - Sedentary life style

Management
- Acute MI management (give at initial presentation): For both ST segment elevation MI and acute coronary syndrome (unstable angina or non-ST segment elevation MI)
  - Bedrest with continuous ECG monitoring.
  - Oxygen to maintain saturation > 90%.
  - ASA ± clopidogrel (*Plavix*) and an anticoagulant (see **Table 14**).
  - If catheterization with angioplasty/stent placement is planned, give a glycoprotein IIb/IIIa inhibitor (see **Table 14**).

- Nitroglycerin is indicated acutely for persistent ischemia, hypertension, large anterior infarction, or HF. Begin at 5–10 μg/min IV and titrate to pain relief, SBP > 90 mm Hg, or resolution of ECG abnormalities.
- Morphine sulfate 1–5 mg IV if chest pain persists on nitroglycerin therapy.
- β-Blockers given acutely and continued chronically unless systolic failure or pronounced bradycardia is present. Acute phase: Atenolol (*Tenormin*) 5 mg IV over 5 min and repeat in 10 min, or metoprolol (*Lopressor*) 5 mg IV q 5 min up to a total of 15 mg. Begin chronic phase within 1–2 h: atenolol 25–100 mg po qd or metoprolol 50–200 mg po bid.

Table 14. Antithrombotic Therapy in Acute Coronary Syndrome		
Class, Agent	**Dosage**	**Indications in Acute Coronary Syndrome**
Antiplatelet Agents		
ASA	162–325 mg po initially followed by 75–160 mg po qd	PACS, DACS, PCI, CABG
Clopidogrel (*Plavix*)	300 mg po initially followed by 75 mg po qd	DACS, PCI*
Anticoagulants		
Enoxaparin (*Lovenox*)	30 mg IV bolus, followed by 1 mg/kg SC q 12 h	DACS
Dalteparin (*Fragmin*)	120 IU/kg SC q 12 h	DACS
Heparin (*Hep-Lock*)	60–70 U/kg (maximum 5000 U) IV bolus followed by 12–15 U/kg/h IV	PCI, CABG
Glycoprotein IIb/IIIa Inhibitors		
Abciximab (*ReoPro*)	0.25 mg/kg IV bolus followed by 0.125 μg/kg/min (maximum 10 μg/min)	PCI
Eptifibatide (*Integrilin*)	180 μg/kg IV bolus followed by 2.0 μg/kg/min IV	PCI
Tirofiban (*Aggrastat*)	0.4 μg/kg/min IV for 30 min, followed by 0.1 μg/kg/min	PCI

Note: PACS = possible or suspected acute coronary syndrome; DACS = definite acute coronary syndrome; PCI = acute coronary syndrome with planned percutaneous cardiac intervention; CABG = acute coronary syndrome with emergent CABG a likely possibility
*Use clopidogrel in PACS if patient is allergic to ASA. In combination with ASA, clopidogrel causes increased risks of bleeding, so use carefully in the elderly. Do not use clopidogrel if there is a reasonable possibility that patient will be undergoing CABG within the next 5 d.

- Thrombolytic therapy for Q-wave MI (chest pain < 12 h, $\geq$ 1 mm ST-segment elevation):
  - Age is not a contraindication.
  - Absolute contraindications (ACC/AHA):

    o Prior hemorrhagic stroke
    o Other stroke or intracerebral event in past yr
    o Active internal bleeding

    o Known intracranial neoplasm
    o Aortic dissection

- Relative contraindications:
  - BP >180/110 on presentation
  - Hx of prior stroke or known intracerebral pathology not covered in absolute contraindications
  - Current therapeutic INR ≥ 3
  - Known bleeding diathesis
  - Recent (< 3 wk) major surgery
  - Prolonged (>10 min) or traumatic CPR
  - Recent (< 2–4 wk) trauma or internal bleeding
  - Noncompressible vascular puncture
  - Active peptic ulcer
  - Hx of severe, chronic HTN
  - For streptokinase or anistreplase, prior exposure (5 d–2 yr) or prior allergic reactions
- Intervention: Percutaneous transluminal coronary angioplasty (PTCA), preferably with stent placement, or emergent coronary artery bypass grafting (CABG) are alternatives to thrombolytic therapy.
- Subacute pharmacologic management (give during hospitalization): For both ST-segment elevation MI and acute coronary syndrome (unstable angina or non-Q-wave MI)
  - Patients with hematocrit ≤ 30 and who are not in HF should be transfused to achieve hematocrit > 33.
  - ACE inhibitors should be started within first 24 h following MI with ST-segment elevation, particularly in cases with systolic dysfunction, eg: captopril (*Capoten*), 6.25–25 mg po bid–tid; enalapril (*Vasotec*), 2.5–20 mg po qd/bid; lisinopril (*Prinivil*, *Zestril*), 2.5–20 mg po qd. Start at low dose and titrate to maximum tolerated dose.
  - Warfarin therapy is indicated in post-MI patients with atrial fibrillation, left ventricular thrombosis, or large anterior infarction (see **Table 10**).
  - Lipid-lowering therapy (see Dyslipidemia section, p 28) to achieve target levels (total cholesterol < 160 mg/dL, LDL cholesterol < 100 mg/dL, HDL cholesterol > 45 mg/dL) should be initiated by the time of hospital discharge.
  - At time of discharge, prescribe rapid-acting nitrates prn: Sublingual nitroglycerin or nitroglycerin spray every 5 min for maximum of 3 doses in 15 min. See **Table 15**.
  - Longer-acting nitrates should be prescribed if symptomatic angina and treatment will be medical rather than surgical or angioplasty. May be combined with β-blockers or calcium channel blockers, or both. See **Table 15**.
  - Calcium channel blockers should be used cautiously for management of angina only in non-Q-wave infarctions without systolic dysfunction and a contraindication to β-blockers.

Table 15. Nitrate Dosages and Formulations		
Drug	**Dosage**	**Formulations**
Oral		
Isosorbide dinitrate (*Isordil, Sorbitrate*)	10–40 mg tid (6 h apart)	T: 5, 10, 20, 30, 40; CT: 5, 10
Isosorbide dinitrate SR (*Isordil Tembids, Dilatrate SR*)	40–80 mg bid–tid	T: 40
Isosorbide mononitrate (*ISMO, Monoket*)	20 mg bid (8 AM and 3 PM)	T: 10, 20
Isosorbide mononitrate SR (*Imdur*)	start 30–60 mg qd; max 240 mg/d	T: 30, 60, 120
Nitroglycerin (*Nitro-Bid*)	2.5–9 mg bid–tid	T: 2.5, 6.5, 9

(*continues*)

Table 15. Nitrate Dosages and Formulations (cont.)		
Drug	Dosage	Formulations
Sublingual		
Isosorbide dinitrate (*Isordil, Sorbitrate*)	1 tablet prn	T: 2.5, 5, 10
Nitroglycerin (*Nitrostat*)	0.4 mg prn	T: 0.15, 0.3, 0.4, 0.6
Oral spray		
Nitroglycerin (*Nitrolingual*)	1–2 spr prn; max 3/15 min	0.4 mg/spr
Ointment		
Nitroglycerin 2% (*Nitro-Bid, Nitrol*)	start 0.5–4 inches q 4–8 h	2%
Transdermal		
Nitroglycerin (*Deponit*) (*Minitran*) (*Nitrek*) (*Nitro-Our*) (*Nitrodisc*) (*Transderm-Nitro*)	1 pat 12–14 h/d	0.2, 0.4 (mg/h) 0.1, 0.2, 0.4, 0.6 0.2, 0.4, 0.6 (mg/h) 0.1, 0.2, 0.3, 0.4, 0.6, 0.8 0.2, 0.3, 0.4 0.1, 0.2, 0.4, 0.6, 0.8

POST MI AND CHRONIC STABLE ANGINA CARE

- Unless contraindicated, all patients should be on ASA, a β-blocker, and an ACE inhibitor.
- If β-blockers are contraindicated, use long-acting nitrates or long-acting calcium channel blockers for chronic angina.
- Use sublingual or spray nitroglycerin for acute angina.
- Treat hypertension; goal of < 140/90 or < 130/80 if HF, diabetes, or renal failure is present.
- Treat dyslipidemia; goals of LDL < 100 mg/dL and TG < 150 mg/dL.
- Treat diabetes; see p 55 for target goals.
- Weight reduction in obese individuals; goal BMI < 25 kg/m^2.
- Aerobic exercise; goal 30 min at least 3 times/wk.
- Smoking cessation.
- Use folic acid 1 mg po qd to treat homocysteinemia; goal homocysteine < 10 μmoles/L.
- Increase consumption of oily fish (eg, white canned or fresh tuna, salmon, mackerel, herring) and foods rich in α-linolenic acid (eg, flax seed, canola, and soybean oils; flaxseed; walnuts). Consider supplementation with fish oil capsules to achieve omega-3 fatty acid intake of 1 g/d.
- Strongly consider placement of implantable cardiac defibrillator in patients with LVEF ≤ 30% at least 1 mo after MI or 3 mo after CABG.

HEART FAILURE
Evaluation and Assessment
- All patients initially presenting with HF should have an echocardiogram to evaluate left ventricular function. An ejection fraction (EF) of < 40% indicates systolic dysfunction. Heart failure with an EF ≥ 40% indicates diastolic dysfunction.

- Other routine assessment tests: ECG, CXR, CBC, electrolytes, creatinine, albumin, LFTs, TSH, UA
- Measurement of plasma brain natriuretic peptide (BNP) can be helpful in diagnosing acute heart failure. A BNP > 100 pg/mL strongly suggests decreased LV function or acute HF.
- Optional: Radionuclide ventriculography, which measures EF more precisely, provides a better evaluation of right ventricular function, and is more expensive than echocardiography

Table 16. Heart Failure Staging		
Clinical Profile	ACC/AHA Staging	New York Heart Association Staging
Asymptomatic but at high risk for developing HF (eg, HTN, diabetes mellitus, CAD present)	Stage A	—
Asymptomatic with structural disease: LVH, left ventricular dysfunction, prior MI, or valvular disease	Stage B	Class I
Structural disease; currently asymptomatic but with hx of symptoms	Stage C	Class I
Structural disease; patient comfortable at rest but symptomatic on normal physical activity	Stage C	Class II
Structural disease; patient comfortable at rest but symptomatic on slight physical activity	Stage C	Class III
Structural disease; patient symptomatic at rest	Stage C	Class IV
Refractory symptoms at rest in hospitalized patient requiring specialized interventions or hospice care	Stage D	Class IV

Management*
Nonpharmacologic:
- Exercise: Regular walking or cycling for NYHA Class I–III or AHA/ACC Stage A–C disability (See **Table 16**)
- Measure weight daily
- Salt restriction: 3 g sodium diet is reasonable goal; 2 g in severe HF
Pharmacologic: For information on drug dosages and side effects not listed below, see **Table 18**. Clinicians should be aware that efficacy of different medications may vary significantly across racial and ethnic groups; eg, African-Americans may require higher doses of ACE inhibitors and β-blockers.
- Systolic dysfunction:
  - Diuretics if volume overload
  - ACE inhibitors to target levels, eg, 150 mg/d of captopril or > 20 mg/d of enalapril or lisinopril
  - For all stable patients with little or no fluid retention, a β-blocker (metoprolol XL [*Toprol-XL*] 12.5–25 mg po qd initially, maximum 200 mg/d; or bisoprolol [*Zebeta*] 1.25 mg po qd initially, maximum 5 mg qd); or carvedilol (*Coreg*) 3.125 mg po bid initially, maximum 25 mg bid should be added for long-term HF management if there is no contraindication to β-blockers (do not add β-blockers in acutely ill patients).
  - Add low-dose digoxin (*Lanoxin*) [T: 0.125, 0.25; S: 0.05 mg/mL]; (*Lanoxicaps*) [T: 0.05, 0.1, 0.2], 0.125–0.375 mg qd (target serum levels 0.5–0.8 mg/dL) if HF is not controlled

on diuretics and ACE inhibitors. Digoxin may be less effective and even harmful in women.
- For patients with NYHA Class III or IV failure and creatinine < 2.5 mg/dL, addition of spironolactone (*Aldactone*) 25 mg qd [T: 25] can reduce mortality; follow serum potassium.
- For patients with MI in the previous 2 wk, LVEF < 40%, and Cr < 2.5 mg/dL, addition of eplerenone (*Inspra*) 25–50 mg po qd [T: 25, 50, 100] can reduce morbidity and mortality; monitor serum potassium.
- An angiotensin II receptor blocker is indicated in patients being treated with a diuretic, a β-blocker, and digoxin and who cannot receive an ACE inhibitor secondary to cough or angioedema.
- Some clinicians recommend anticoagulating patients with EF < 25% (see **Table 10**).
- Calcium channel blockers, Class I antiarrhythmics, hydralazine, and nitroglycerin are not indicated.
• Diastolic dysfunction:
- Diuretics should be used judiciously and only if there is volume overload.
- There is no agreed-upon treatment of diastolic dysfunction. β-Blockers, ACE inhibitors, and/or non-dihydropyridine calcium channel blockers may be of benefit.

*Source: Hunt SA, Baker DW, Chin MH, et al. ACC/AHA guidelines for the evaluation and management of chronic heart failure in the adult: executive summary: a report of the American College of Cardiology/American Heart Association Task Force on Practice Guidelines (Committee to Revise the 1995 Guidelines for Evaluation and Management of Heart Failure). *Circulation* 2001;104:2996–3007.

DYSLIPIDEMIA
Treatment Indications
• Treat dyslipidemia if overt atherosclerotic disease: CHD (angina, previous MI), peripheral arterial disease, abdominal aortic aneurysm, or symptomatic carotid artery disease (TIA or prior stroke). Treatment goal is LDL < 100 mg/dL.
• National Cholesterol Education Program recommends treating diabetes mellitus as CHD risk equivalent. Treatment goal is LDL < 100 mg/dL.
• Consider dyslipidemia treatment in older adults without overt atherosclerotic disease or diabetes, but with multiple other CHD risk factors (HTN, smoking, family hx of premature CHD, HDL < 40 mg/dL, male sex). In general, treatment goals are LDL < 130 mg/dL for 2+ risk factors and < 160 mg/dL for 0–1 risk factors. However, more severe individual risk factor profiles may indicate the need for a lower LDL level treatment goal. See www.nhlbi.nih.gov.

Management
Nonpharmacologic: A cholesterol-lowering diet should be considered initial therapy for dyslipidemia and should be used as follows:
• The patient should be at low risk for malnutrition.
• The diet should be nutritionally adequate, with sufficient total calories, protein, calcium, iron, and vitamins.
• The diet should be easily understood and affordable (a dietitian can be very helpful).
• Cholesterol-lowering margarines can lower LDL cholesterol by 10% to 15% (*Take Control* 1–2 tablespoons/d; *Benecol* 3 servings of 1.5 teaspoons each/d).
Pharmacologic: Target drug treatment according to type of dyslipidemia.

Table 17. Drug Regimens for Dyslipidemia			
Condition	**Drug**	**Dosage**	**Formulations**
Elevated LDL, normal TG	HMG-CoA reductase inhibitor*		
	Atorvastatin (*Lipitor*)	10–80 mg qd	T: 10, 20, 40, 80
	Fluvastatin (*Lescol*)	20–80 mg qd in PM, max 80 mg	C: 20, 40; T: ER 80
	Lovastatin (*Mevacor*)	10–80 mg qd–bid	T: 10, 20, 40
	Pravastatin (*Pravachol*)	10–40 mg qd	T: 10, 20, 40, 80
	Rosuvastatin (*Crestor*)	10–40 mg qd	T: 5, 10, 20, 40
	Simvastatin (*Zocor*)	5–80 mg qd in PM	T: 5, 10, 20, 40, 80
Elevated TG (> 500 mg/dL)	Gemfibrozil (*Lopid*)	300–600 mg po bid	T: 600
Combined elevated LDL, low HDL, elevated TG	Gemfibrozil, HMG-CoA (if TG < 300 mg/dL)	as above	as above
Alternative for any of above	Niacin†	100 mg tid to start; increase to 500–1000 mg tid; extended release 150 mg qhs to start, increase to 2000 mg qhs as needed	T: 25, 50, 100, 250, 500, ER 150, 250, 500, 750, 1000; C: TR 125, 250, 400, 500
Elevated LDL or combined with inadequate response to one agent	Lovastatin/niacin combination*† (*Advicor*)	20 mg/500 mg qhs to start; increase to 40 mg/ 2000 mg as needed	T: 20/500, 20/750, 20/1000
	Colesevelam (*WelChol*)	Monotherapy: 1850 mg po bid; combination therapy: 2500–3750 mg/d in single or divided doses	T: 625
	Ezetimibe (*Zetia*)	10 mg qd	T: 10

* Baseline CPK and transaminases. Repeat CPK if symptoms of myopathy. Repeat transaminases at 3 mo, then periodically. Watch for myopathy at higher doses or when used with another antidyslipidemic drug. Should be taken in the evening.
† Monitor for flushing, pruritus, nausea, gastritis, ulcer. Dosage increases should be spaced 1 mo apart. ASA 325 mg po 30 min before first niacin dose of the day is quite effective in preventing side effects.

HYPERTENSION
Definition, Classification
JNC 7 defines HTN as SBP > 140 or DBP > 90. In elderly persons, base treatment decisions primarily on the SBP level.

Evaluation and Assessment
• Measure both standing and sitting BP after 5 min of rest.
• Base diagnosis on two or more readings at each of two or more visits. Once diagnosis is made, evaluation includes:
  - Assessment of cardiac risk factors: smoking, dyslipidemia, obesity, and diabetes mellitus are important in older adults.

- Assessment of end-organ damage: LVH, angina, prior MI, prior coronary revascularization, HF, stroke or TIA, nephropathy, peripheral arterial disease, retinopathy.
- Routine laboratory tests: CBC, UA, electrolytes, creatinine, fasting glucose, total cholesterol, HDL cholesterol, and ECG.
- Think renal artery stenosis if sudden onset of HTN, sudden rise in BP in previously well-controlled HTN, or HTN despite treatment with three antihypertensives.

Aggravating Factors

Almost all are related to life style:

- Emotional stress
- Excessive alcohol intake
- Excessive salt intake
- Lack of aerobic exercise
- Low potassium intake
- Low calcium intake
- Nicotine
- Obesity

Management

(JNC 7 recommendations.) Target is < 140/90 (130/80 in persons with diabetes or kidney disease). Lowering BP below 120/80 is not recommended.

Nonpharmacologic:

- Adequate calcium and magnesium intake as well as a low-fat diet are recommended for optimizing general health.
- Adequate dietary potassium intake; fruits and vegetables are the best sources.
- Aerobic exercise—30–45 min most days of the week—is recommended.
- Moderation of alcohol intake—limit to 1 oz of ethanol/d.
- Moderation of dietary sodium: watch for volume depletion with diuretic use. Goal: 2.4 g Na^+/d.
- Smoking cessation
- Weight reduction in obese persons: even a 10-lb weight loss can significantly lower BP. Goal: BMI < 25 kg/m^2.

Pharmacologic:

Table 18 lists commonly used antihypertensives.

- Use antihypertensives carefully in patients with orthostatic BP drop.
- Base treatment decisions on standing BP.
- In the absence of coexisting conditions, a thiazide diuretic, a β-blocker, or an ACE inhibitor can be used as a first-line drug.
- In the presence of coexisting conditions, therapy should be individualized (see **Table 19**).
- Combination drugs for hypertension are listed in **Table 20**.
- Available dose formulations of oral potassium supplements: [T: (mEq) 6, 7, 8, 10, 20; S: (mEq/15 mL) 20, 40; powders (mEq/pk) l5, 20, 25]
- Follow-up BP measurements monthly until target BP is attained; visits may be q 3–6 mo if BP is stable at target goal.

Hypertensive Emergencies and Urgencies:

- Elevated BP alone without symptoms or target end organ damage rarely requires emergent BP lowering.
- Conditions requiring emergent BP lowering include hypertensive encephalopathy, intracranial hemorrhage, unstable angina, acute MI, acute LV failure with pulmonary edema, dissecting aortic aneurysm.

- Most common initial treatment for emergent BP lowering is sodium nitroprusside (*Nipride*) 0.25–10 mg/kg/min as IV infusion.
- For nonemergent (ie, urgent) BP lowering, give a standard dose of a recommended antihypertensive orally (see **Table 18**) or an extra dose of the patient's usual oral antihypertensive.

Class, Drug	Geriatric Dosage Range, total mg/d (times/d)	Formulations	Comments (Metabolism, Excretion)
Diuretics			↓ potassium, Na, magnesium levels; ↑ uric acid, calcium, cholesterol (mild), and glucose (mild) levels
Thiazides			
√ Chlorothiazide (*Diuril*)	125–500 (1)	T: 250, 500	
√ Chlorthalidone (*Hygroton*)	12.5–25 (1)	T: 15, 25, 50, 100	↑ side effects at > 25 mg/d (L)
√ HCTZ (*Esidrix, HydroDIURIL, Oretic*)	12.5–25 (1)	T: 25, 50, 100; S: 50 mg/mL; C: 12.5	↑ side effects at > 25 mg/d (L)
√ Indapamide (*Lozol*)	0.625–2.5 (1)	T: 1.25, 2.5	Less or no hypercholesterolemia (L)
√ Metolazone (*Mykrox*)	0.25–0.5 (1)	T rapid: 0.5	Monitor electrolytes carefully (L)
√ Metolazone (*Zaroxolyn*)	2.5–5 (1)	T: 2.5, 5, 10	Monitor electrolytes carefully (L)
√ Polythiazide (*Renese*)	1–4 (1)	T: 1, 2, 4	
Loop diuretics			
♥ Bumetanide (*Bumex*)	0.5–4 (1–3)	T: 0.5, 1, 2	Short duration of action, no hypercalcemia (K)
♥ Furosemide (*Lasix*)	20–160 (1–2)	T: 20, 40, 80; S: 10, 40 mg/5 mL	Short duration of action, no hypercalcemia (K)
♥ Torsemide (*Demadex*)	2.5–50 (1–2)	T: 5, 10, 20, 100	Short duration of action, no hypercalcemia (K)
Potassium-sparing drugs			
Amiloride (*Midamor*)	2.5–10 (1)	T: 5	(L, K)
Triamterene (*Dyrenium*)	25–100 (1–2)	T: 50, 100	(L, K)
Aldosterone receptor-blockers			Useful in certain cases of heart failure (see p 28)
♥ Eplerenone (*Inspra*)	25–100 (1)	T: 25, 50, 100	(L, K)
♥ Spironolactone (*Aldactone*)	12.5–50 (1–2)	T: 25, 50, 100	Gynecomastia (L, K)
Adrenergic Inhibitors			
α_1-Blockers			Avoid as primary therapy for HTN unless patient has BPH

Note: Listing of side effects is not exhaustive, and side effects are for the class of drugs except where noted for individual drugs. √ = preferred for treating older persons; ♥ = useful in treating heart failure.

(*continues*)

Table 18. Oral Antihypertensive Agents (cont.)			
Class, Drug	Geriatric Dosage Range, total mg/d (times/d)	Formulations	Comments (Metabolism, Excretion)
Doxazosin (*Cardura*)	1–16 (1)	T: 1, 2, 4, 8	(L)
Prazosin (*Minipress*)	1–20 (2–3)	T: 1, 2, 5	(L)
Terazosin (*Hytrin*)	1–20 (1–2)	T: 1, 2, 5, 10; C: 1, 2, 5, 10	(L, K)
Central α_2-Agonists and other Centrally Acting Drugs			Sedation, dry mouth, bradycardia, withdrawal hypertension
Clonidine (*Catapres, Catapres-TTS*)	0.1–1.2 (2–3) *or* 1 patch/wk	T: 0.1, 0.2, 0.3; patch: 0.1, 0.2, 0.3 mg/d	(L, K)
Guanfacine (*Tenex*)	0.5–2 (1)	T: 1, 2	(K)
Methyldopa (*Aldomet*)	250–2500 (2)	T: 125, 250, 500; S: 250 mg/5 mL	(L, K)
Reserpine (*Serpasil*)	0.05–0.25 (1)	T: 0.1, 0.25	Depression, nasal congestion, activation of peptic ulcer (L, K)
β-Blockers			Bronchospasm, bradycardia, acute heart failure, may mask insulin-induced hypoglycemia; lipid solubility is a risk factor for delirium
√ Acebutolol (*Sectral*)	200–800 (1)	C: 200, 400	β_1, low lipid solubility, intrinsic sympathomimetic activity (L, K)
√ Atenolol (*Tenormin*)	12.5–100 (1)	T: 25, 50, 100	β_1, low lipid solubility (K)
√ Betaxolol (*Kerlone*)	5–20 (1)	T: 10, 20	β_1, low lipid solubility (L, K)
√ ♥ Bisoprolol (*Zebeta*)	2.5–10 (1)	T: 5, 10	β_1, low lipid solubility (L, K)
√ Carteolol (*Cartrol*)	1.25–10 (1)	T: 2.5, 5	β_1, low lipid solubility, intrinsic sympathomimetic activity (K)
√ Metoprolol (*Lopressor*)	25–400 (2)	T: 25, 50, 100	β_1, moderate lipid solubility (L)
√ ♥ Long-acting (*Toprol XL*)	50–400 (1)	T: 25, 50, 100, 200	(L)
Nadolol (*Corgard*)	20–160 (1)	T: 20, 40, 80, 120, 160	β_1, β_2, low lipid solubility (K)
Penbutolol (*Levatol*)	10–40 (1)	T: 20	β_1, β_2, high lipid solubility, intrinsic sympathomimetic activity, (L, K)
Pindolol (*Visken*)	5–40 (2)	T: 5, 10	β_1, β_2, moderate lipid solubility, intrinsic sympathomimetic activity (K)
Propranolol (*Inderal*)	20–160 (2)	T: 10, 20, 40, 60, 80, 90; S: 4 mg/mL, 8 mg/mL, 80 mg/mL	β_1, β_2, high lipid solubility (L)

Note: Listing of side effects is not exhaustive, and side effects are for the class of drugs except where noted for individual drugs. √ = preferred for treating older persons; ♥ = useful in treating heart failure.

Class, Drug	Geriatric Dosage Range, total mg/d (times/d)	Formulations	Comments (Metabolism, Excretion)
Table 18. Oral Antihypertensive Agents (cont.)			
Long-acting (*Inderal LA, Innopran XL*)	60–180 (1)	C: 60, 80, 120, 160	β_1, β_2, high lipid solubility (L)
Timolol (*Blocadren*)	10–40 (2)	T: 5, 10, 20	β_1, β_2, low to moderate lipid solubility (L, K)
Combined α- and β-Blockers			Postural hypotension, bronchospasm
√ ♥ Carvedilol (*Coreg*)	3.125–25 (2)	T: 3.125, 6.25, 12.5, 25	β_1, β_2, high lipid solubility (L)
√ Labetalol (*Normodyne, Trandate*)	100–600 (2)	T: 100, 200, 300	β_1, β_2, moderate lipid solubility (L, K)
Direct Vasodilators			Headaches, fluid retention, tachycardia
Hydralazine (*Apresoline*)	25–100 (2–4)	T: 10, 25, 50, 100	Lupus syndrome (L, K)
Minoxidil (*Loniten*)	2.5–50 (1)	T: 2.5, 10	Hirsutism (K)
Calcium Antagonists			
Nondihydropyridines			Conduction defects, worsening of systolic dysfunction, gingival hyperplasia
√ Diltiazem SR (*Cardizem CD, Cardizem SR, Dilacor XR, Tiazac*)	120–360 (1–2) max 480	C: 1/d: 120, 180, 240, 300, 360, 420; 2/d: 60, 90, 120; T: 30, 60, 90, 120, ER: 120, 180, 240	Nausea, headache (L)
√ Verapamil SR (*Calan SR, Covera-HS, Isoptin SR, Verelan*)	120–360 (1–2)	T: SR 120, 180, 240; C: SR 100, 120, 180, 200, 240, 300, 360; T: 40, 80, 120	Constipation, bradycardia (L)
Dihydropyridines			Ankle edema, flushing, headache, gingival hypertrophy
√ Amlodipine (*Norvasc*)	2.5–10 (1)	T: 2.5, 5, 10	(L)
√ Felodipine (*Plendil*)	2.5–20 (1)	T: 2.5, 5, 10	(L)
√ Isradipine (*DynaCirc*)	2.5–20 (2)	T: 2.5, 5	(L)
√ Sustained release (*DynaCirc CR*)	2.5–10 (1)	T: 5, 10	
√ Nicardipine (*Cardene*)	60–120 (3)	C: 20, 30	(L)
√ Sustained release (*Cardene SR*)	60–120 (2)	T: 30, 45, 60	(L)
√ Nifedipine SR (*Adalat CC, Procardia XL*)	30–60 (1)	T: 30, 60, 90	(L)
√ Nisoldipine (*Sular*)	10–40 (1)	T: ER 10, 20, 30, 40	(L)

Note: Listing of side effects is not exhaustive, and side effects are for the class of drugs except where noted for individual drugs. √ = preferred for treating older persons; ♥ = useful in treating heart failure.

(*continues*)

Table 18. Oral Antihypertensive Agents (cont.)			
Class, Drug	Geriatric Dosage Range, total mg/d (times/d)	Formulations	Comments (Metabolism, Excretion)
ACE Inhibitors			Cough (common), angioedema (rare), hyperkalemia, rash, loss of taste, leukopenia
√ ♥ Benazepril (*Lotensin*)	2.5–40 (1–2)	T: 5, 10, 20, 40	(L, K)
√ ♥ Captopril (*Capoten*)	12.5–150 (2–3)	T: 12.5, 25, 50, 100	(L, K)
√ ♥ Enalapril (*Vasotec*)	2.5–40 (1–2)	T: 2.5, 5, 10, 20	(L, K)
√ ♥ Fosinopril (*Monopril*)	5–40 (1–2)	T: 10, 20, 40	(L, K)
√ ♥ Lisinopril (*Prinivil, Zestril*)	2.5–40 (1)	T: 2.5, 5, 10, 20, 30, 40	(K)
√ ♥ Moexipril (*Univasc*)	3.75–30 (1)	T: 7.5, 15	(L, K)
√ ♥ Perindopril (*Aceon*)	4–8 (1–2)	T: 2, 4, 8	(L, K)
√ ♥ Quinapril (*Accupril*)	5–40 (1)	T: 5, 10, 20, 40	(L, K)
√ ♥ Ramipril (*Altace*)	1.25–20 (1)	T: 1.25, 2.5, 5, 10	(L, K)
√ ♥ Trandolapril (*Mavik*)	1–4 (1)	T: 1, 2, 4	(L, K)
Angiotensin II Receptor Blockers (ARBs)			Angioedema (very rare), hyperkalemia
√ ♥ Candesartan (*Atacand*)	4–32 (1)	T: 4, 8, 16, 32	(K)
√ ♥ Eprosartan (*Teveten*)	400–800 (1–2)	T: 400, 600	(biliary, K)
√ ♥ Irbesartan (*Avapro*)	75–300 (1)	T: 75, 150, 300	(L)
√ ♥ Losartan (*Cozaar*)	12.5–100 (1–2)	T: 25, 50, 100	(L, K)
√ ♥ Olmesartan (*Benicar*)	20–40 (1)	T: 5, 20, 40	(F, K)
√ ♥ Telmisartan (*Micardis*)	20–80 (1)	T: 20, 40, 80	(L)
√ ♥ Valsartan (*Diovan*)	40–320 (1)	T: 80, 160, 320; C: 80, 160	(L, K)

Note: Listing of side effects is not exhaustive, and side effects are for the class of drugs except where noted for individual drugs. √ = preferred for treating older persons; ♥ = useful in treating heart failure.
Source: Data in part from the seventh report of the Joint National Committee on Prevention, Detection, Evaluation, and Treatment of High Blood Pressure: the JNC 7 report. *JAMA.* 2003;289:2560–2572.

Table 19. Choosing Antihypertensive Therapy on the Basis of Coexisting Conditions		
Condition	Appropriate For Use	Avoid or Contraindicated
Angina	β, D, non-D	
Atrial tachycardia and fibrillation	β, non-D	
Bronchospasm		β, $\alpha\beta$
Diabetes mellitus	ACEI, ARB, β, T†	T‡
Dyslipidemia		β, T‡
Essential tremor	β	
HF	AA, ACEI, ARB, β, $\alpha\beta$, L	D, non-D*
Hyperthyroidism	β	
MI	β, AA, ACEI	non-D

Table 19. Choosing Antihypertensive Therapy on the Basis of Coexisting Conditions (cont.)		
Condition	Appropriate For Use	Avoid or Contraindicated
Osteoporosis	T	
Prostatism (BPH)	α	
Renal insufficiency	AA, ACEI§	
Urge UI	D, non-D	L, T

Note: AA = aldosterone antagonist; α = α-blocker; β = β-blocker; $\alpha\beta$ = combined α- and β-blocker; ACEI = ACE inhibitor; ARB = angiotensin receptor blocker; D = dihydropyridine calcium antagonist; L = loop diuretic; non-D = nondihydropyridine calcium antagonist; T = thiazide diuretic.

* May be beneficial in HF caused by diastolic dysfunction.

† Low-dose diuretics are probably beneficial in type 2 diabetes; high-dose diuretics are relatively contraindicated in types 1 and 2.

‡ Low-dose diuretics have a minimal effect on lipids.

§ Use with great caution in renovascular disease.

Table 20. Combination Drugs for Hypertension		
Combination Type	Fixed-dose Combination, mg*	Trade Name
ACE inhibitors and calcium channel blockers	Amlodipine/benazepril hydrochloride (2.5/10, 5/10, 5/20, 10/20)	*Lotrel*
	Enalapril maleate/felodipine (5/5)	*Lexxel*
	Trandolapril/verapamil (2/180, 1/240, 2/240, 4/240)	*Tarka*
ACE inhibitors and diuretics	Benazepril/HCTZ (5/6.25, 10/12.5, 20/12.5, 20/25)	*Lotensin HCT*
	Captopril/HCTZ (25/15, 25/25, 50/15,50/25)	*Capozide*
	Enalapril maleate/HCTZ (5/12.5, 10/25)	*Vaseretic*
	Lisinopril/HCTZ (10/12.5, 20/25)	*Prinzide*
	Moexipril hydrochloride/HCTZ (7.5/12.5, 15/25)	*Uniretic*
	Quinapril hydrochloride/HCTZ (10/12.5, 20/12.5, 20/25)	*Accuretic*
Angiotensin-receptor blockers and diuretics	Candesartan cilexetil/HCTZ (16/12.5, 32/12.5)	*Atacand HCT*
	Eprosartan mesylate/HCTZ (600/12.5, 600/25)	*Teveten HCT*
	Irbesartan/HCTZ (75/12.5, 150/12.5, 300/12.5)	*Avalide*
	Losartan potassium/HCTZ (50/12.5, 100/25)	*Hyzaar*
	Telmisartan/HCTZ (40/12.5, 80/12.5)	*Micardis HCT*
	Valsartan/HCTZ (80/12.5, 160/12.5)	*Diovan HCT*
β-Blockers and diuretics	Atenolol/chlorthalidone (50/25, 100/25)	*Tenoretic*
	Bisoprolol fumarate/HCTZ (2.5/6.25, 5/6.25, 10/6.25)	*Ziac*
	Propranolol LA/HCTZ (40/25, 80/25)	*Inderide*
	Metoprolol tartrate/HCTZ (50/25, 100/25)	*Lopressor HCT*
	Nadolol/bendroflumethiazide (40/5, 80/5)	*Corzide*
	Timolol maleate/HCTZ (10/25)	*Iimolide*
Centrally acting drug and diuretic	Methyldopa/HCTZ (250/15, 250/25, 500/30, 500/50)	*Aldoril*
	Reserpine/chlorothiazide (0.125/250, 0.25/500)	*Diupres*
	Reserpine/HCTZ (0.125/25, 0.125/50)	*Hydropres*
Diuretic and diuretic	Amiloride hydrochloride/HCTZ (5/50)	*Moduretic*
	Spironolactone/HCTZ (25/25, 50/50)	*Aldactazide*
	Triamterene/HCTZ (37.5/25, 50/25, 75/50)	*Dyazide, Maxzide*

* Some drug combinations are available in multiple fixed doses. Each drug dose is reported in mg.

Source: The seventh report of the Joint National Committee on Prevention, Detection, Evaluation, and Treatment of High Blood Pressure: the JNC 7 report. *JAMA.* 2003;289:2560–2572.

ATRIAL FIBRILLATION
Evaluation and Assessment
Causes:
- Cardiac disease: Cardiac surgery, cardiomyopathy, HF, hypertensive heart disease, ischemic disease, pericarditis, valvular disease
- Noncardiac disease: Alcoholism, chronic pulmonary disease, infections, pulmonary emboli, thyrotoxicosis

Standard testing: ECG, CXR, CBC, electrolytes, creatinine, BUN, TSH, echocardiogram

Management
- Correct precipitating cause(s).
- Acute-onset:
  - D/C cardioversion if compromised cardiac output or angina
  - If hemodynamically stable with rapid ventricular response (> 100 beats/min), lower ventricular rate medically. Options include:
    - β-Blockers (eg, atenolol [*Tenormin*] 5 mg IV over 5 min, may repeat in 10 min [0.5 mg/mL], followed by 25–100 mg po qd [T: 25, 50, 100]);
    - Calcium channel blockers (eg, diltiazem [*Cardizem injectable*] 20 mg IV bolus, giving 25 mg IV 15 min later if necessary, with a maintenance infusion of 5–15 mg/h, followed by 120–360 mg po qd of long-acting preparation [*Cardizem CD, Dilacor XR*; T: 120, 180, 240, 300, 360].
    - Digoxin [*Lanoxin*] is another option, although it works more slowly for rate control: 0.25 mg IV q 6 h up to 0.75 mg [0.05 mg/mL], followed by 0.125–0.25 mg po qd [T: 0.125, 0.25].
  - If electric cardioversion or lowering of ventricular rate has not converted patient to sinus rhythm, begin anticoagulation with IV unfractionated heparin followed by oral warfarin (see p 17); seek cardiology consultation for possible electric or pharmacologic cardioversion.
- Chronic AF:
  - Anticoagulate (see **Table 10**) if there are no contraindications.
  - If anticoagulation is contraindicated, begin ASA 325 mg po qd.
  - If electric cardioversion has not been tried in the past, seek cardiology consultation for possible cardioversion.
  - Rate control (goal < 80/min averaged over 1 h) can be achieved with oral β-blockers, calcium channel blockers, or digoxin (see above for examples and dosages).

AORTIC STENOSIS (AS)
Evaluation and Assessment
- Presence of symptoms—angina, syncope, HF (frequently diastolic dysfunction)—indicates severe disease and a life expectancy without surgery of < 2 yr.
- Echocardiography is essential in the work-up to measure aortic jet velocity (AJV) and aortic valve area (AVA).
  - Moderate AS is indicated by an AJV of 3.0–4.0 meters/sec and by an AVA of 1.0–1.5 cm^2.
  - Severe AS is indicated by an AJV > 4.0 meters/sec and by an AVA < 1.0 cm^2.

- For asymptomatic cases, echocardiography should be repeated annually for moderate AS and every 6–12 mo for severe AS.
- ECG and CXR should be obtained initially to look for conduction defects, LVH, and pulmonary congestion.

Treatment
- Aortic valve replacement (AVR) surgery
  - Alleviates symptoms and improves ventricular functioning.
  - In most cases, perform AVR promptly *after* symptoms have appeared.
  - Consider risks and benefits of AVR on individual basis (see pp 131–133).
- There is no effective medical treatment. Avoid vasodilators if possible.

PERIPHERAL ARTERIAL DISEASE

Table 21. Classes of Peripheral Arterial Disease			
Class	ABI	Symptoms	Treatment
Normal	> 0.9	None	RFM
Mild	0.8–0.9	No limitation in walking distance	RFM, AT
Moderate to severe	0.4–0.8	Walking limited by claudication	RFM, AT, CRx
Severe to critical	< 0.4	Rest pain; ischemia on exam	RFM, AT, CRx, LS

Note: ABI = ankle-brachial BP index; AT = antiplatelet therapy; CRx = claudication therapy; LS = limb salvage; RFM = risk factor modification.

Treatment
Risk Factor Modification:
- Low-fat diet
- Exercise: walking program
- Smoking cessation
- Lipid-lowering therapy
- BP control
- Glycemic control in diabetic patients

Antiplatelet Therapy:
- ASA 325 mg qd
- Clopidogrel (*Plavix*) 75 mg qd [T: 75] if ASA failure or intolerant to ASA

Claudication Treatment:
- Walking program
- Drug therapy: cilostazol (*Pletal*) 100 mg bid (contraindicated in patients with HF) 1 h before or 2 h after meals [T: 50, 100]; pentoxifylline (*Trental*) 400 mg tid [T: 400]; conventional analgesics

Limb Salvage:
- Percutaneous angioplasty
- Bypass surgery

SYNCOPE

Table 22. Classification of Syncope			
Cause	Frequency (%)	Features	Increased Risk of Death
Vasovagal	21	Preceded by lightheadedness, nausea, diaphoresis; recovery gradual, frequently with fatigue	No
Cardiac	10	Little or no warning before blackout, rapid and complete recovery	Yes
Orthostatic	9	Lightheaded prodrome after standing, recovery gradual	No
Medication-induced	7	Lightheaded prodrome, recovery gradual	No
Seizure	5	No warning, may have neurologic deficits, slow recovery	Yes
Stroke/TIA	4	Little or no warning, neurologic deficits	Yes
Other causes	8	Preceded by cough, micturition, or specific situation	No
Unknown	37	Any of the above	Yes

Source: Adapted from Soteriades ES, Evans JC, Larson MG, et al. Incidence and prognosis of syncope. *N Engl J Med* 2002;347:878–885.

Evaluation
- Focus hx on events before, during, and after loss of consciousness; hx of cardiac disease (significantly worsens prognosis of syncope of all causes); careful medication review.
- Focus on cardiovascular and neurologic systems in physical examination.
- ECG and orthostatic BP/pulse check for all patients.
- Additional testing as suggested initial evaluation:
  - Ambulatory ECG monitoring for further evaluation of arrhythmia
  - Stress testing to investigate ischemic heart disease
  - Echocardiography to investigate structural heart disease
  - Electrophysiologic studies in patients with prior MI and structural heart disease
  - Tilt-table testing for suspected vasovagal cause
  - Head imaging, electroencephalogram for suspected neurologic cause
  - If suspected orthostatic cause, evaluation for Parkinson's disease, autonomic neuropathy, diabetes mellitus, hypovolemia

Management
- Patients with cardiac syncope require immediate hospitalization on telemetry; exclude MI and PE.
- Strongly consider hospital admission for patients with syncope due to neurologic or unknown causes, particularly if concurrent heart disease.
- Patients with syncope due to vasovagal, orthostatic, medication-induced, or other causes can usually be managed as outpatients, particularly if there is no hx of heart disease.
- Treatment is correction of underlying cause.

DIAGNOSIS
Diagnostic Criteria—Adapted from *DSM-IV*
- Disturbed consciousness (ie, decreased attention, environmental awareness)
- Cognitive change (eg, memory deficit, disorientation, language disturbance), or perceptual disturbance (eg, visual illusions, hallucinations)
- Rapid onset (hours to days) and fluctuating daily course
- Evidence of a causal physical condition

Risk Factors
- Dementia greatly increases risk for delirium.
- Advanced age, comorbid physical problems (especially sleep deprivation, immobility, dehydration, pain, sensory impairment).

Evaluation
- Assume reversibility unless proven otherwise.
- Thoroughly review prescription and OTC medications.
- Exclude infection and other medical causes.
- Laboratory studies may include CBC, electrolytes, LFTs, renal function tests, serum calcium and glucose, UA, oxygen saturation, CXR, and ECG
- Confusion Assessment Method (CAM): BOTH acute onset and fluctuating course AND inattention AND EITHER disorganized thinking OR altered level of consciousness (Inouye S, *Ann Intern Med.* 1990;113:941–948).

CAUSES
(Italicized type indicates the most common causes in older persons.)
Drugs
- *Anticholinergics* (eg, diphenhydramine), TCAs, (eg, amitriptyline, imipramine), antipsychotics (eg, chlorpromazine, thioridazine)
- Anti-inflammatory agents, including prednisone
- Benzodiazepines or alcohol—acute toxicity or withdrawal
- Cardiovascular (eg, digitalis, antihypertensives)
- Diuretics
- Lithium
- GI (eg, cimetidine, ranitidine)
- Opioid analgesics (especially meperidine)

Infections
Respiratory, skin, urinary tract, and others

Metabolic Disorders
Acute blood loss, *dehydration, electrolyte imbalance*, end-organ failure (hepatic, renal), hyperglycemia, *hypoglycemia, hypoxia*

Cardiovascular
Arrhythmia, *HF, MI*, shock

Neurologic
CNS infections, head trauma, seizures, stroke, subdural hematoma, TIAs, tumors

Miscellaneous
Fecal impaction, *postoperative state*, sleep deprivation, urinary retention

MANAGEMENT

Nonpharmacologic
- Identify and remove or treat underlying cause(s)
- Provide general supportive measures:
  - Environmental modifications
    - communication to reorient to new surroundings
    - objects that provide orientation (eg, calendar, clock)
    - quiet, well-lit surroundings
    - familiar faces (eg, family members) at bedside for reassurance
    - sitters
  - Stimulating activities during daytime
    - cognitive activities (eg, current events discussion, word games)
    - ambulation, active range-of-motion exercises
  - Correction of sensory deficits
    - eyeglasses
    - adequate lighting
    - magnifying lenses
    - cerumen removal
    - hearing aids
    - portable amplification device
  - Measures to promote normal sleep
    - warm milk at bedtime
    - relaxation tapes
    - back massage
    - nighttime noise reduction
  - Prevention of dehydration
    - oral or parenteral supplementation if BUN/creatinine ratio > 18
  - Physical restraints (only as last resort to maintain patient safety, eg, preventing patient from pulling out tubes or catheters)

Pharmacologic
- For acute agitation or aggression accompanying delirium, use a high-potency antipsychotic such as haloperidol (*Haldol*) 0.5–2 mg po [T: 0.5, 1, 2, 5, 10, 20; S: 2 mg/mL] or IV or IM (twice as potent as po). May also be given as slow IV push; titrate upward as needed. Reevaluate every 30 min. Observe for development of EPS. Ziprasidone (*Geodon*) also available IM, but concerns about cardiac conduction delays limit use for this indication. Avoid low-potency antipsychotics such as chlorpromazine (*Thorazine*) or thioridazine (*Mellaril*) because of their anticholinergic and arrythmogenic properties (torsade de pointes). If patient is able to take drugs po, consider low dose of atypical antipsychotic (see **Table 64**).
- If delirium is secondary to alcohol or benzodiazepine withdrawal, use a benzodiazepine such as lorazepam (*Ativan*) in doses of 0.5–2 mg every 4–6 h. Since these agents themselves may cause delirium, gradual withdrawal and discontinuation are desirable. If delirium is secondary to alcohol, also use thiamine 100 mg qd (po, IM, or IV).

DEMENTIA

DEMENTIA SYNDROME
Definition
Acquired decline in memory and in at least one other cognitive function (eg, language, visual-spatial, executive) sufficient to affect daily life in an alert person.

Estimated Frequencies of Dementia Causes
- AD: 60% to 70%
- Other progressive disorders: 15% to 30% (eg, vascular, Lewy body)
- Completely reversible dementia (eg, drug toxicity, metabolic changes, thyroid disease, subdural hematoma, normal-pressure hydrocephalus): 2% to 5%

DIAGNOSIS OF AD
- Dementia syndrome
- Gradual onset and continuing decline
- Not due to another physical, neurologic, or psychiatric condition or to medications
- Deficits not occurring exclusively during delirium

PROGRESSION OF AD
Mild Cognitive Impairment   (preclinical)   MMSE: 26–30
- Delayed paragraph recall
- Cognition otherwise intact
- No functional impairment
- Mild construction, language, or executive dysfunction
- Some cases of mild cognitive impairment may not progress to AD

Early, Mild Impairment   (yr 1–3 from onset of symptoms)   MMSE: 22–28
- Disorientation for date
- Naming difficulties (anomia)
- Recent recall problems
- Mild difficulty copying figures
- Decreased insight
- Social withdrawal
- Irritability, mood change
- Problems managing finances

Middle, Moderate Impairment   (yr 2–8)   MMSE: 10–21
- Disoriented to date, place
- Comprehension difficulties (aphasia)
- Impaired new learning
- Getting lost in familiar areas
- Impaired calculating skills
- Delusions, agitation, aggression
- Not cooking, shopping, banking
- Restless, anxious, depressed
- Problems with dressing, grooming

Late, Severe Impairment   (yr 6–12)   MMSE: 0–9
- Nearly unintelligible verbal output
- Remote memory gone
- Unable to copy or write
- No longer grooming or dressing
- Incontinent
- Motor or verbal agitation

NONCOGNITIVE SYMPTOMS
Psychotic Symptoms (eg, Delusions, Hallucinations)
• Occur in about 20% of AD patients
• Delusions may be paranoid (eg, people stealing things, spouse unfaithful)
• Hallucinations (approximately 11% of patients) are more commonly visual

Depressive Symptoms
• Occur in up to 40% of AD patients; may herald onset of AD
• May cause acceleration of decline if untreated
• Need to suspect if patient stops eating or withdraws

Agitation or Aggression
• Occurs in up to 80% of patients with AD
• A leading cause of nursing-home admission
• Consider superimposed delirium or pain as a trigger

RISK AND PROTECTIVE FACTORS FOR AD

Definite Risks	Possible Risks	Possible Protections
Age	Other genes	Antioxidants (eg, vitamin E, beta carotene)
Family history	Head trauma	
Down syndrome	Lower educational level	
APOE-E4	Depression	

Clinical Features Distinguishing AD and Other Types of Dementia
• AD: Memory, language, visual-spatial disturbances, indifference, delusions, agitation
• Frontotemporal dementia: Personality change, executive dysfunction, hyperorality, relative preservation of visual-spatial skills
• Lewy body dementia: visual hallucinations, delusions, extrapyramidal symptoms, fluctuating mental status, sensitivity to antipsychotic medications

EVALUATION
Although completely reversible (eg, drug toxicity) dementia is rare, identifying and treating secondary physical conditions may improve function.
• History: Obtain from family or other informant
• Physical and neurologic examination
• Assess functional status
• Evaluate mental status for attention, immediate and delayed recall, remote memory, executive function, and depression. Screening tests may include Mini-Cog (p 183), number of animals named in 1 min, MMSE, GDS (p 185)

Laboratory Testing
CBC, TSH, B_{12}, serum calcium, liver and renal function tests, electrolytes, serologic test for syphilis (selectively); at this time genetic testing and commercial "Alzheimer blood tests" are not recommended for clinical use.

Neuroimaging
The likelihood of detecting structural lesions is increased with:
• Onset age < 60
• Focal (unexplained) neurologic signs or symptoms

• Abrupt onset or rapid decline (weeks to months)
• Predisposing conditions (eg, metastatic cancer or anticoagulants)

Neuroimaging may detect the 5% of patients with clinically significant structural lesions that would otherwise be missed.

TREATMENT

Primary goals of treatment are to improve quality of life and maximize functional performance by enhancing cognition, mood, and behavior.

General Treatment Principles

• Identify and treat comorbid physical illnesses (eg, HTN, diabetes mellitus)
• Avoid anticholinergic medications, eg, benztropine, diphenhydramine, hydroxyzine, oxybutynin, TCAs, clozapine, thioridazine
• Set realistic goals
• Limit prn psychotropic medication use
• Specify and quantify target behaviors
• Maximize and maintain functioning

Nonpharmacologic Approaches

To improve function:
• Behavior modification, scheduled toileting, and prompted toileting (see p 171) for UI
• Graded assistance (as little help as possible to perform ADLs), practice, and positive reinforcement to increase independence

For problem behaviors:
• Music during meals, bathing
• Walking or light exercise
• Simulate family presence with video or audio tapes
• Pet therapy
• Speak at patient's comprehension level
• Bright light, white noise

Pharmacologic Treatment of Cognitive Dysfunction in AD

• Patients with a diagnosis of mild or moderate AD should receive a cholinesterase inhibitor that will increase level of acetylcholine in brain (**Table 23**) (demonstrated benefit for cognition, mood, behavioral symptoms, and daily function). Controlled data show benefits of cholinergic drugs for 1 yr and open trials demonstrate benefit for 3 yr. Only 25% of patients taking cholinesterase inhibitors show clinical improvement but 80% have less rapid decline. Initial studies show benefits of these drugs for patients with Lewy body dementia and dementia with vascular risk factors. Cholinergic therapy may attenuate noncognitive symptoms and delay nursing-home placement. To evaluate response or stabilize:
  - Elicit caregiver observations of patient's behavior (alertness, initiative) and follow functional status (ADLs and IADLs).
  - Follow cognitive status (eg, improved or stabilized) by caregiver's report or serial ratings of cognition (eg, Mini-Cog, see p 183; MMSE).
• Consider the antioxidant vitamin E at 1000 IU bid (shown to delay functional decline thought to occur from oxidative stress).

- *Ginkgo biloba* is not generally recommended because clinical trial results are not yet definitive, and preparations vary because such nutriceuticals are not FDA regulated (see **Table 8**).
- Estrogen replacement therapy in older women may increase risk of developing AD.

Table 23. Cognitive Enhancers		
Drug	**Formulations**	**Dosing (Metabolism)**
Donepezil (*Aricept*)*	T: 5, 10	Start at 5 mg qd, increase to 10 mg qd after 1 mo (CYP2D6, 3A4) (L)
Galantamine (*Reminyl*)*	T: 4, 8, 12; S: 4 mg/mL	Start at 4 mg bid, increase to 8 mg bid after 4 wk; recommended dose 16–24 mg/d (CYP2D6, 3A4) (L)
Rivastigmine (*Exelon*)*	T: 1.5, 3, 4.5, 6	Start at 1.5 mg bid and gradually titrate up to 6 mg bid as tolerated; retitrate if drug is stopped (K)
Memantine (*Namenda* [NMDA antagonist])	T: 5, 10	Start at 5 mg qd, increase by 5 mg at weekly intervals to maximum of 10 mg bid

* Cholinesterase inhibitors. Side effects increase with higher dosing. Continue if improvement or stabilization occurs; stopping drugs can lead to rapid decline. Possible side effects include nausea, vomiting, diarrhea, dyspepsia, anorexia, weight loss, leg cramps, bradycardia, insomnia, and agitation.

Treatment of Agitation

Table 24. Agitation Treatment Guidelines			
Symptom	**Drug**	**Dosage**	**Formulations**
Agitation in context of nonacute psychosis	Risperidone* (*Risperdal*)	0.25–1.5 mg/d	T: 0.25, 0.5, 1, 2, 3, 4; S: 1 mg/mL
	Olanzapine (*Zyprexa*) (*Zydis*)	2.5–10 mg/d	T: 2.5, 5, 7.5, 10, 15, 20 T: orally disintegrating 5, 10, 15, 20
	Quetiapine (*Seroquel*)	25–400 mg/d	T: 25, 100, 200, 300
Acute psychosis agitation if IM or IV is needed	Haloperidol (*Haldol*)	0.5–2 mg/d**	T: 0.5, 1, 2, 5, 10, 20; S: 2 mg/mL; Inj
Agitation in context of depression	SSRI, eg, citalopram (*Celexa*)	10–30 mg/d	T: 20, 40; S: 2 mg/mL
Anxiety, mild to moderate irritability	Trazodone (*Desyrel*)	50–100 mg/d†	T: 50, 100, 150, 300
	Buspirone (*BuSpar*)	30–60 mg/d‡	T: 5, 7.5, 10, 15, 30
As a possible second-line treatment for significant agitation or aggression	Divalproex sodium (*Depakote*)	500–1500 mg/d§	T: 125, 250, 500; S: syr 250 mg/mL; sprinkle capsule: 125
	Carbamazepine (*Tegretol*)	300–600 mg/d§§	T: 200; ChT: 100; S: sus 100/5 mL

Table 24. Agitation Treatment Guidelines (cont.)			
Symptom	**Drug**	**Dosage**	**Formulations**
Sexual aggression, impulse-control symptoms in men	Estrogen (*Premarin*) or medroxyprogesterone (*Depo-Provera*)	0.625–1.25 mg/d 100 mg IM/wk	T: 0.3, 0.625, 0.9, 1.25, 2.5 Inj

* Use with caution in patients with cerebrovascular disease or hypovolemia; may increase risk of cerebrovascular adverse events compared with placebo; similar comparative data not available for other atypical antipsychotics.
** May need to give higher doses in emergency situations; should be used for only short periods of time.
† Small divided daytime dosage and larger bedtime dosage; watch for sedation and orthostasis.
‡ Can be given bid; 2–4 wk for adequate trial.
§ Can monitor serum levels; usually well tolerated; check CBC, platelets for agranulocytosis, thrombocytopenia risk in older patients.
§§ Monitor serum levels; periodic CBCs, platelet counts secondary to agranulocytosis risk. Beware of drug-drug interactions.

CAREGIVER ISSUES
- Over 50% develop depression.
- Physical illness, isolation, anxiety, and burnout are common.
- Intensive education and support of caregivers may delay institutionalization.
- Adult day care for patients and respite services may help.
- Alzheimer's Association offers support, education; chapters are located in major cities throughout US. (See p 203 for telephone, Web site.)
- Family Caregiver Alliance offers support, education, information for caregivers. (See p 203 for telephone, Web site.)

ADDITIONAL REFERENCES
Doody RS, Stevens JC, Beck C, et al. Practice parameter: management of dementia (an evidence-based review): report of the Quality Standards Subcommittee of the American Academy of Neurology. *Neurology* 2001; 56(9):1154–1166.

Palmer K, Fratiglioni L, Winblad B. What is mild cognitive impairment? Variations in definitions and evolution of nondemented persons with cognitive impairment. *Acta Neuro Scand.* 2003;107(Suppl 179):14–20.

EVALUATION AND ASSESSMENT

Recognizing and diagnosing late-life depression can be difficult. Older patients may complain of lack of energy or other somatic symptoms, attribute symptoms to old age or other physical conditions, or fail to mention them to a health care professional.

Medical Evaluation

TSH, B$_{12}$, calcium, LFTs, renal function tests, electrolytes, UA, CBC

DSM-IV Criteria for Major Depressive Episode (Abbreviated)

Five or more of the following symptoms have been present during the same 2-wk period and represent a change from previous functioning; at least one of the symptoms is either (1) depressed mood or (2) loss of interest or pleasure.

- Depressed mood
- Loss of interest or pleasure in activities
- Significant weight loss or gain (not intentional), or decrease or increase in appetite
- Insomnia or hypersomnia
- Psychomotor agitation or retardation
- Fatigue or loss of energy
- Feelings of worthlessness or excessive or inappropriate guilt
- Diminished ability to think or concentrate, or indecisiveness
- Recurrent thoughts of death, suicidal ideation, attempt, or plan

The *DSM-IV* criteria are not specific for older adults; cognitive symptoms may be more prominent. The GDS and other instruments are useful for screening and monitoring (see p 185).

MANAGEMENT

Treatment should be individualized on the basis of hx, past response, and severity of illness as well as concurrent illnesses. Treatments may be combined.

Nonpharmacologic

For mild to moderate depression or in combination with pharmacotherapy: cognitive-behavioral therapy, interpersonal therapy, problem-solving therapy.

Pharmacologic

For mild, moderate, or severe depression: the duration of therapy should be at least 6–12 mo following remission for patients experiencing their first depressive episode. Most older patients with a hx of major depression require lifelong antidepressant therapy.

Choosing an Antidepressant (see Table 25 and list at top of p 49)

First-line Therapy: Consider an SSRI for most older patients, especially those with:

- Heart conduction defects or ischemic heart disease
- Prostatic hyperplasia
- Uncontrolled glaucoma

Second-line Therapy: Consider venlafaxine, mirtazapine, or bupropion
Third-line Therapy: Consider nortriptyline or desipramine for patients with:
- Severe melancholic depression
- Urge incontinence, but use tolterodine (*Detrol*) and an SSRI if avoidance of central anticholinergic effects of a TCA is important (see **Table 79**)

Bupropion, T$_3$, methylphenidate, olanzapine, or risperidone may be useful augmentation to SSRI in cases of partial response. Quetiapine, olanzapine, or risperidone, or electroconvulsive therapy may be necessary for psychotic depression.

Table 25. Antidepressants Used for Older Adults				
Class, Drug	Initial Dosage	Usual Dosage	Formulations	Comments (Metabolism, Excretion)
Selective Serotonin-Reuptake Inhibitors				Class side effects (EPS, hyponatremia) (L, K [10%])
Citalopram (*Celexa*)	10–20 mg qam	20–30 mg/d	T: 20, 40, 60; S: 5 mg/ 10 mL	
Escitalopram (*Lexapro*)	10 mg/d	10 mg/d	T: 5, 10, 20	Currently limited geriatric experience
Fluoxetine (*Prozac*)	5 mg qam	5–60 mg/d	T: 10; C: 10, 20, 40; S: 20 mg/5 mL; C: SR 90 (weekly dose)	Long half-lives of parent and active metabolite may allow for less frequent dosing; may cause more insomnia than other SSRIs; CYP2D6, -2C9, -3A4 inhibitor (L)
Fluvoxamine (*Luvox*)	25 mg qhs	100–300 mg/d	T: 25, 50, 100	Not approved as an antidepressant in US; CYP1A2, -3A4 inhibitor (L)
Paroxetine (*Paxil*)	5 mg	10–40 mg/d	T: 10, 20, 30, 40	Helpful if anxiety symptoms are prominent; increased risk of withdrawal symptoms (dizziness); CYP2D6 inhibitor (L)
(*Paxil CR*)	12.5 mg/d	—	T: ER 12.5, 25, 37.5; S: 10 mg/5 mL	Increase by 12.5 mg/d no faster than 1/wk
Sertraline (*Zoloft*)	25 mg qam	50–200 mg/d	T: 25, 50, 100; S: 20 mg/mL	(L)
Additional Medications				
Bupropion (*Wellbutrin, Zyban*)	37.5–50 mg bid 100 mg (SR) qd or bid	75–150 mg bid 100–150 mg (SR) bid	T: 75, 100, SR 100, 150	Consider for SSRI, TCA nonresponders; safe in HF; may be stimulating; can lower seizure threshold (L) *(continues)*

Table 25. Antidepressants Used for Older Adults (cont.)				
Class, Drug	Initial Dosage	Usual Dosage	Formulations	Comments (Metabolism, Excretion)
Methylphenidate (*Ritalin*)	2.5–5 mg at 7 AM and noon	5–10 mg at 7 AM and noon	T: 5, 10, 20	Short-term treatment of depression or apathy in physically ill elderly; used as an adjunct (L)
Mirtazapine (*Remeron*)	15 mg qhs	15–45 mg/d	T: 15, 30, 45	May increase appetite; sedating; oral disintegrating tablet (SolTab) available (L)
Nefazodone (*Serzone*)	50 mg bid	200–400 mg/d	T: 50, 100, 150, 200, 250	May help insomnia; sedating in some patients; CYP3A4 inhibition; hepatoxicity, obtain baseline LFT (L)
Trazodone (*Desyrel*)	25 mg qhs	75–600 mg/d	T: 50, 100, 150, 300	Sedation may limit dose; may be used as a hypnotic; ventricular irritability; priapism in men (L)
Venlafaxine (*Effexor*)	25–50 mg bid	75–225 mg/d	T: 25, 37.5, 50, 75, 100	Low anticholinergic activity; minimal sedation and hypotension; may increase BP; may be useful when somatic pain present; EPS, withdrawal symptoms, hyponatremia (L)
(*Effexor XR*)	75 mg qam	75–225 mg/d	C: 37.5, 75, 150	Same as above
Tricyclic Antidepressants				
Desipramine (*Norpramin*)	10–25 mg qhs	50–150 mg/d	T: 10, 25, 50, 75, 100, 150	Therapeutic serum level >115 ng/mL (L)
Nortriptyline (*Aventyl, Pamelor*)	10–25 mg qhs	75–150 mg/d	C: 10, 25, 50, 75; S: 10 mg/ 5 mL	Therapeutic window (50–150 ng/mL) (L)
Monoamine Oxidase Inhibitors				Hypotension; drug, food interactions (K, L)
Isocarboxazid (*Marplan*)	10 mg bid–tid	10 mg tid	T: 10	
Phenelzine (*Nardil*)	15 mg qd	15–60 mg/d	T: 15	
Tranylcypromine (*Parnate*)	10 mg bid	20–40 mg/d	T: 10	

Antidepressants to Avoid in Older Adults
- Amitriptyline (eg, *Elavil*): anticholinergic, sedating, hypotensive
- Amoxapine (*Asendin*): anticholinergic, sedating, hypotensive; also associated with EPS, tardive dyskinesia, and neuroleptic malignant syndrome
- Doxepin (eg, *Sinequan*): anticholinergic, sedating, hypotensive
- Imipramine (*Tofranil*): anticholinergic, sedating, hypotensive
- Maprotiline (*Ludiomil*): seizures and rashes
- Protriptyline (*Vivactil*): very anticholinergic; can be stimulating
- St. John's wort: decreases effects of digoxin and CYP3A4 substrates; efficacy questioned
- Trimipramine (*Surmontil*): anticholinergic, sedating, hypotensive

Electroconvulsive Therapy
Generally safe and very effective.
Indications: Severe depression when a rapid onset of response is necessary; when depression is resistant to drug therapy; for patients who are unable to tolerate antidepressants, have previous response to ECT, have psychotic depression, severe catatonia, or depression with Parkinson's disease.
Complications: Temporary confusion, arrhythmias, aspiration, falls.
Contraindications:
- Increased intracranial pressure
- Intracranial tumor
- MI within 3 mo (relative)
- Stroke within 1 mo (relative)

Before ECT evaluation: CXR, ECG, serum electrolytes, and cardiac examination. Additional tests (eg, stress test, neuroimaging, EEG) are used selectively.

DERMATOLOGIC CONDITIONS

COMMON DERMATOLOGIC CONDITIONS

Table 26. Dermatologic Conditions Common in Elderly Persons

Condition	Areas Affected	Description
Candidiasis	Body folds	Erythema, pustules, or cheesy, whitish matter, satellite lesions
Treatment: See intertrigo, next; antifungal powders (see list in next section)		
Intertrigo	Any place 2 skin surfaces rest against one another (eg, under the breasts)	Moist, erythematous with local superficial skin loss; satellite lesions due to candida
Treatment: Keep area dry; topical antifungals (see list in next section), absorbent pwd, 1% hydrocortisone or 0.1% triamcinolone crm bid × 1 or 2 d if inflamed		
Neurodermatitis	Any skin surfaces	Generalized, localized itching
Treatment: Mid- to higher-potency topical corticosteroids (**Table 27**); exclude other causes		
Onychomycosis	Nails	Thickening and discoloration
Treatment: Itraconazole (*Sporanox*)—toenails: 200 mg po qd × 3 mo or 200 mg po bid × 1 wk/mo × 3 mo; fingernails: 200 mg po bid × 1 wk/mo × 2 mo (L); fluconazole (*Diflucan*)—toenails: 150 or 300 mg po/wk × 6–12/mo; fingernails: 150 or 300 mg po/wk × 3–6 mo (L); terbinafine (*Lamisil*)—toenails: 250 mg po qd × 12 wk; fingernails: 250 mg qd × 6 wk. Obtain nail specimens for laboratory culturing to confirm diagnosis before prescribing itraconazol or terbinafine		
Psoriasis	All skin areas, nails (pitting)	Well-defined, erythematous plaques covered with silver scales; severity varies
Treatment: Topical corticosteroids, UV light, PUVA, methotrexate, cyclosporine, etretinate, sulfasalazine; anthralin preparations and tar + 1% to 4% salicylic acid; calcipotriene for nonfacial areas		
Rosacea	Face (nose, chin, cheeks, forehead)	Vascular and follicular dilation; mild to moderate
Treatment: Avoid triggers (stress, prolonged sun exposure and exercise, alcohol, hot drinks, spicy foods). Wear sun screen. Topical: azelaic acid 15% gel bid (*Finacea*) or 20% crm bid (*Azelax, Finevin*); metronidazole 0.75% crm or gel bid (*Metrocream, Metrogel*) or 1% crm qd (*Naritate*); sodium sulfacetamide 10% + sulfa 5% qd (*Rosula* aqueous gel, *Clenia* crm, foaming wash), avoid if sulfa allergy or kidney disease (K) Oral: tetracycline 500 mg bid–tid, doxycycline 100 mg qd, minocycline 100 mg bid, clarithromycin 250–500 mg bid		
Scabies	Interdigital webs, flexor aspects of wrists, axillary, umbilicus, nipples, genitals	Burrows, erythematous papules or nodules, dry or scaly skin, pruritus
Treatment: Can result in epidemics; treat all contacts and treat environment. Apply topical products from head to toe: Permethrin (*Elimite*) 5% crm q 8–14 h, remove; crotamiton (*Eurax*) 10% crm × 24 h, repeat, then cleansing bath in 48 h; or 1% lindane (*K-well, Scabene*) crm q 8–12 h, remove; oatmeal baths, topical corticosteroids, or emollient creams for symptom relief; ivermectin (*Stromectol*) 200 µg/kg orally; may repeat once in 1 or 2 wk [T: 3, 6]		

Table 26. Dermatologic Conditions Common in Elderly Persons (cont.)		
Condition	Areas Affected	Description
Seborrheic dermatitis	Nasal labial folds, eyebrows, hairline, sideburns, posterior auriculare and midchest	Greasy, yellow scales with or without erythematous base; common in Parkinson's disease and in debilitated patients
Treatment: Hydrocortisone 1% crm bid or triamcinolone 0.1% oint bid × 2 wk; scalp: shp (selenium sulfide, zinc, or tar); ketoconazole 2% crm for severe conditions when infection from *Pityrosporum orbiculare* is suspected		
Skin maceration	Any area constantly in contact with moisture, covered with occlusive dressing or bandage; skin folds, groin, buttocks	Erythema; abraded, excoriated skin; blisters; white and silver patches
Treatment: Eliminate cause of moisture: toileting program for incontinence; condom catheter; indwelling catheter (reserve for most intractable conditions); fecal incontinence collector. Protect skin from moisture: clean gently with mild soap after each incontinent episode; apply moisture barrier (eg, *Vaseline, Proshield, Smooth and Cool, Calmoseptene*) to repel moisture; use disposable briefs that wick moisture from the skin; use linen incontinence pads when disposable briefs accentuate perineal dermatitis.		
Urticaria		
Hives	Skin surface	Uniform, red edematous plaques surrounded by white halos
Treatment: Identify cause, oral H₁ antihistamines (see **Table 67**), oral glucocorticoids (eg, prednisone 40 mg qd), oral H₂ antihistamines, or doxepin (po or topical *Zonalon 5%*) for refractory cases.		
Angioedema	Lips, eyelids, tongue, larynx, GI tract	Larger, deeper than hives
Treatment: Oral H₁ antihistamines (see **Table 67**), oral glucocorticoids. Severe reactions: SC epinephrine 0.3 mL of a 1:1000 dilution (*EpiPen*)		
Cholinergic	Skin surface	Round, red papular wheals
Treatment: Oral H₁ antihistamines (see **Table 67**) 1 h before exercise. Hot shower may relieve itching.		
Xerosis	All skin surfaces	Dull, rough, flaky, cracked; nummular
Treatment: ↑ Humidity, apply emollient oint (eg, *Aquaphor*) or crm (eg, *Eucerin*) immediately after bathing; oatmeal baths; hydrocortisone 1% oint; avoid excess bathing and bath oils (falls)		

DERMATOLOGIC MEDICATIONS

Topical Antifungals

- Amphotericin B (*Fungizone*) [3% crm, lot, or oint]
- Clotrimazole (*Lutrimin, Mycelex*) [1% crm, lot, sol]
- Econazole nitrate (*Spectazole*) [1% crm]
- Ketoconazole (*Nizoral*) [2% crm or shp]
- Miconazole (eg, *Monistat-Derm*) [2% crm, lot, pwd, spr, tinc]
- Nystatin (*Mycostatin, Nilstat, Nystex*) [100,000 units/g crm, oint, pwd]
- Terbinafine (*Lamisil*–OTC) [1% crm, gel]

Oral Antifungals
- Fluconazole (*Diflucan*) [T: 50, 100, 150, 200; S: 10, 40 mg/mL]
- Itraconazole (*Sporonax*) [C: 100; S: 100 mg/mL]
- Terbinafine (*Lamisil*) [T: 250]

Table 27. Topical Corticosteroids		
Name	**Strength and Formulations**	**Frequency of Application**
Lowest Potency		
Dexamethasone phosphate (*Decaderm*)	0.1% crm	qd–qid
Hydrocortisone acetate (*Hytone*)	0.25%, 0.5%, 1%, 2.5% crm, oint	tid–qid
Low Potency		
Alclometasone dipropionate (*Aclovate*)	0.05% crm, oint	bid–tid
Betamethasone valerate (*Valisone*)	0.1% lot	bid–qid
Desonide (*DesOwen, Tridesilon*)	0.05% crm, lot, oint	bid–qid
Fluocinolone acetonide (*Synalar*)	0.025% crm, 0.01% sol	bid–qid
Triamcinolone acetonide (*Aristocort, Kenalog*)	0.1% crm, 0.025% crm, lot, oint	bid–tid
Mid-potency		
Betamethasone dipropionate (*Diprosone*)	0.05% lot	bid–qid
Betamethasone valerate (*Valisone*)	0.1% crm	bid–qid
Clocortolone pivalate (*Cloderm*)	0.1% crm	qd–qid
Desoximetasone (*Topicort*)	0.05% crm	bid
Fluocinolone acetonide (*Synalar*)	0.025% crm, oint	bid–qid
Flurandrenolide (*Cordran*)	0.05% crm, oint, lot	qd–bid
Fluticasone propionate (*Cutivate*)	0.05% crm	bid
Hydrocortisone butyrate (*Locoid*)	0.1% crm	qd–bid
Hydrocortisone valerate (*Westcort*)	0.2% crm, oint	tid–qid
Mometasone furoate (*Elocon*)	0.1% crm, lot	qd
Prednicarbate (*Dermatop*)	0.1% crm, lot	bid
Triamcinolone acetonide (*Aristocort, Kenalog*)	0.1% lot, oint	bid–tid
High Potency		
Amcinonide (*Cyclocort*)	0.1% crm, lot	bid–tid
Betamethasone dipropionate (*Diprosone*)	0.05% crm	bid–qid
Betamethasone valerate (*Valisone*)	0.01% oint	bid–qid
Diflorasone diacetate (*Florone, Maxiflor*)	0.05% crm	bid–qid
Fluocinonide (*Lidex-E*)	0.05% crm	bid–qid
Fluticasone propionate (*Cutivate*)	0.005% oint	bid
Triamcinolone acetonide (*Aristocort, Kenalog*)	0.5% oint	bid–tid
Higher Potency		
Amcinonide (*Cyclocort*)	0.1% oint	bid–tid
Betamethasone dipropionate (*Diprolene AF*)	0.05% augmented crm	bid–qid
Betamethasone dipropionate (*Diprosone*)	0.05% oint	bid–qid
Desoximetasone (*Topicort*)	0.25% crm, oint; 0.05% gel	bid
Diflorasone diacetate (*Florone, Maxiflor*)	0.05% oint	bid–qid
Fluocinonide (*Lidex*)	0.05% crm, oint, gel	bid–qid
Halcinonide (*Halog*)	0.1% crm, oint, sol	qd–tid
Mometasone furoate (*Elocon*)	0.1% oint	qd
Super Potency		
Betamethasone dipropionate (*Diprolene*)	0.05% augmented crm, oint	bid–qid
Clobetasol propionate (*Temovate*)	0.05% crm, oint, sol, gel	bid
Diflorasone diacetate (*Psorcon*)	0.05% optimized oint	qd–tid
Halobetasol propionate (*Ultravate*)	0.05% crm, oint	bid

ENDOCRINE DISORDERS

ADRENAL INSUFFICIENCY
Common Causes
- Chronic glucocorticoid administration
- Pituitary tumors
- Tuberculosis
- Autoimmune

Evaluation
- Basal plasma cortisol > 15 μg/dL excludes adrenal insufficiency
- ACTH stimulation test: tetracosactin (*Synacthen Depot*) 250 μg IM or IV; peak value > 19 μg/dL is normal

Pharmacologic Therapy
For corticosteroid dose equivalencies, see **Table 28.**

Management
Stress doses of corticosteroids for patients with severe illness, injury, or undergoing surgery: In emergency situations, do not wait for test results. Give hydrocortisone 100 mg IV q 8 h. For less severe stress, double or triple usual oral replacement dose and taper back to baseline as quickly as possible.

Table 28. Corticosteroids					
Drug	Approx Equivalent Dose (mg)	Relative Anti-Inflammatory Potency	Relative Mineral-ocorticoid Potency	Biologic Half-Life (h)	Formulations
Betamethasone (*Celestone*)	0.6–0.75	20–30	0	36–54	T: 0.6; S: 0.6 mg/5 mL
Cortisone (*Cortone*)	25	0.8	2	8–12	T: 5; S: 50 mg/mL
Dexamethasone (*Decadron, Dexone, Hexadrol*)	0.75	20–30	0	36–54	T: 0.25, 0.5, 0.75, 1, 1.5, 2, 4; S: elixir 0.5 mg/5 mL; Inj
Fludrocortisone (*Florinef*)*	NA	10	4	12–36	T: 0.1
Hydrocortisone (*Cortef, Hydrocortone*)	20	1	2	8–12	T: 5, 10, 20; S: 10 mg/5 mL; Inj
Methylprednisolone (eg, *Medrol, Solu-Medrol, Depo-Medrol*)	4	5	0	18–36	T: 2, 4, 8, 16, 24, 32; Inj
Prednisolone (eg, *Delta-Cortef, Prelone Syr, Pediapred*)	5	4	1	18–36	S: 5 mg/5 mL; syr 5, 15 mg/5 mL
Prednisone (*Deltasone, Liquid Pred, Meticorten, Orasone*)	5	4	1	18–36	T: 1, 2.5, 5, 10, 20, 50; S: 5 mg/5 mL
Triamcinolone (eg, *Aristocort, Kenacort, Kenalog*)	4	5	0	18–36	T: 1, 2, 4, 8; S: syr 4 mg/5 mL

Note: NA = not available.
* Usually given for orthostatic hypotension 0.1 mg qd–tid.

HYPOTHYROIDISM
Common Causes
- Autoimmune (primary thyroid failure)
- Following therapy for hyperthyroidism
- Pituitary or hypothalmic disorders (secondary thyroid failure)
- Medications, especially, amiodarone (rare after first 18 mo of therapy) and lithium

Evaluation
TSH, free T_4

Pharmacologic Therapy
- Thyroxine (T_4, levothyroxine [*Eltroxin, Levo-T, Levothroid, Levoxyl, Synthroid*]). Start 25 μg and increase by 25-μg intervals every 4–6 wk [T: 25, 50, 75, 88, 100, 112, 125, 137, 150, 175, 200, 300 μg].
- Thyroxine and liothyronine (T_3) (*Thyrolar*). Start $^1/_4$ strength and increase [12.5/3.1 ($^1/_4$ strength), 25/6.25 ($^1/_2$ strength), 50/12.5, 100/25, 150/37.5 μg].
- For myxedema coma: Load 400 μg IV or 100 μg q 6–8 h for 1 d, then 100 μg/d for 4 d; then start usual replacement regimen.
- To convert thyroid USP to thyroxine: 60 mg USP = 50 μg thyroxine.
- If patients are npo and must receive IV thyroxine, dose should be half usual po dose.

Monitoring
In primary hypothyroidism, the goal of therapy is to maintain plasma TSH within the normal range. Further adjustments are made every 6–12 wk (12- to 25-μg increments) on basis of TSH levels until TSH is in normal range. Monitor TSH level at least every 12 mo (ATA) in patients on chronic thyroid replacement therapy. Following dose adjustment, recheck TSH in 6–12 wk.

HYPERTHYROIDISM
Common Causes
- Graves' disease
- Toxic nodule
- Toxic multinodular goiter
- Medications, esp. amiodarone (can occur any time during therapy) and lithium

Evaluation
TSH, free T_4. When indicated, T_3, thyroid autoantibodies, radioactive iodine uptake.

Pharmacologic Therapy
- Radioactive iodine ablation is usual treatment of choice, but surgery or medical therapy (see Monitoring above) are options.
- Propylthiouracil (PTU): Start 100 po tid, then adjust up to 200 po tid as needed [T: 50].
- Methimazole (*Tapazole*): Start 5–20 mg po tid, then adjust [T: 5, 10].
- Adjunctive therapy with β-blockers (see **Table 18**) or calcium antagonists (see **Table 18**) may provide symptomatic improvement.

DIABETES MELLITUS
Definition and Classification (ADA)
Diabetes mellitus is a group of metabolic diseases characterized by hyperglycemia resulting from defects in insulin secretion, insulin action, or both.

Type 1: Caused by an absolute deficiency of insulin secretion.

Type 2: Caused by a combination of resistance to insulin action and an inadequate compensatory insulin secretory response.

Criteria for Diagnosis: One or more of the following:
- Symptoms of diabetes (eg, polyuria, polydipsia, unexplained weight loss) plus casual plasma glucose concentration $\geq$ 200 mg/dL
- Fasting (no caloric intake for $\geq$ 8 h) plasma glucose $\geq$ 126 mg/dL
- 2 h Plasma glucose $\geq$ 200 mg/dL during an oral glucose tolerance test (OGTT)

Diagnosis should be confirmed by reevaluating on a subsequent day.

Impaired Fasting Glucose: Defined as fasting plasma glucose $\geq$ 110 and < 126 mg/dL

Impaired Glucose Tolerance: Abnormal casual plasma glucose concentration or response to OGTT but not meeting diagnostic criteria for diabetes

Management
Evaluate for Co-morbid Conditions (AGS): depression (see p 46), polypharmacy (see p 9), cognitive impairment (see p 183), urinary incontinence (see p 170), falls (see p 59), pain (see p 119).

Goals of Treatment (ADA, AGS): Average preprandial capillary blood glucose 80–120 mg/dL, average bedtime capillary blood glucose 100–140 mg/dL, and HbA_{1c} < 7% (ADA); < 8% if frail, life expectancy < 5 yr, or high risk of hypoglycemia, polypharmacy, or drug interaction (AGS).

Nonpharmacologic Interventions:
- Individualized nutrition therapy (see p 92)
- Life style (eg, regular exercise, alcohol and smoking cessation)
- Patient and family education for self-management
- Self-monitoring of blood glucose
- High-fiber diet (25 g insoluble and 25 g soluble/d)

Pharmacologic Interventions for Type 2: Stepped therapy:
1. Monotherapy with a 2nd-generation sulfonylurea agent, metformin, α-glucosidase inhibitor, or thiazolidinedione (see **Table 29**)
2. Combination therapy with 2 or more agents with different actions
3. Add insulin hs or switch to insulin bid (see **Table 30**)

Manage hypertension (BP goal < 130/80 mm Hg; also see p 29) and lipid disorders (p 28; treat as CHD risk equivalent with target LDL < 100 mg/dL, HDL > 40 mg/dL, TG < 150 mg/dL), as appropriate. ACE inhibitor or angiotensin II receptor blocker (ARB) if albuminuria, hypertension, or another cardiovascular risk factor. Check renal function within 1–2 wk of initiation of therapy, with each dose increase, and at least yearly. If ACE inhibitor or ARB is not tolerated, consider nondihydropyridine calcium channel blocker. Daily ASA 81–325 mg.

Table 29. Oral Agents for Treating Diabetes Mellitus

Drug	Dosage	Formulations	Comments (Metabolism)
2nd-Generation Sulfonylureas			Increase insulin secretion; lower HbA_{1c} by 1.0–2.0%
Glimepiride (*Amaryl*)	4–8 mg once, begin 1–2 mg	T: 1, 2, 4	Numerous drug interactions, long-acting (L, K)
Glipizide (generic or *Glucotrol*)	2.5–40 mg once or divided	T: 5, 10	Short-acting (L, K)
(*Glucotrol XL*)	5–20 mg once	T: ER 2.5, 5, 10	Long-acting (L, K)
Glyburide (generic or *Diaβeta, Micronase*)	1.25–20 mg once or divided	T: 1.25, 2.5, 5	Long-acting, risk of hypoglycemia (L, K)
Micronized glyburide (*Glynase*)	1.5–12 mg once	T: 1.5, 3, 4.5, 6	(L, K)
α-Glucosidase Inhibitors			Delay glucose absorption; lower HbA_{1c} by 0.5–1.0%
Acarbose (*Precose*)	50–100 mg tid, just before meals, start with 25 mg	T: 25, 50, 100	GI side effects common, avoid if Cr > 2 mg/dL, monitor LFTs (gut, K)
Miglitol (*Glyset*)	25–100 mg tid, with 1st bite of meal; start with 25 mg qd	T: 25, 50, 100	Same as acarbose but no need to monitor LFTs (L, K)
Biguanides			Decrease hepatic glucose production; lower HbA_{1c} by 1.0–2.0%
Metformin (*Glucophage*) (*Glucophage XR*)	500–2550 mg divided 1500–2000 mg qd	T: 500, 850, 1000 T: ER 500	Avoid in patients > 80 yr, Cr > 1.5 in men, Cr > 1.4 in women, HF, COPD, ↑ LFTs; hold before contrast radiologic studies; may cause weight loss (K)
Meglitinides			Increase insulin secretion; lower HbA_{1c} by 1.0–2.0%
Nateglinide (*Starlix*)	60–120 mg tid	T: 60, 120	Give 30 min before meals
Repaglinide (*Prandin*)	0.5 mg bid–qid if HbA_{1c} < 8% or previously untreated 1–2 mg bid–qid if HbA_{1c} ≥ 8% or previously treated	T: 0.5, 1, 2	Give 30 min before meals, adjust dose at wkly intervals; potential for drug interactions, caution in hepatic, renal insufficiency (L)
Thiazolidinediones			Insulin resistance reducers; lower HbA_{1c} by 0.5–1.0%; ↑ risk of HF; avoid if NYHA Class III or IV cardiac status; D/C if any decline in cardiac status

Table 29. Oral Agents for Treating Diabetes Mellitus (cont.)			
Drug	Dosage	Formulations	Comments (Metabolism)
Pioglitazone (*Actos*)	15 or 30 mg qd; max 45 mg/d as monotherapy, 30 mg/d in combination therapy	T: 15, 30, 45	Check LFTs at start, q 2 mo during 1st yr, then periodically; avoid if clinical evidence of liver disease or if serum ALT levels > 2.5 upper limit of normal (L, K)
Rosiglitazone (*Avandia*)	4 mg qd–bid	T: 2, 4, 8	Check LFTs at start, q 2 mo during 1st yr, then periodically; avoid if clinical evidence of liver disease or if serum ALT levels > 2.5 upper limit of normal (L, K)
Combinations			
Glipizide and metformin (*Metaglip*)	2.5/250 once; 20/2000 in 2 divided doses	T: 2.5/250, 2.5/500, 5/500	Avoid in patients > 80 yr, Cr > 1.5 in men, Cr > 1.4 in women; see individual drugs (L, K)
Glyburide and metformin (*Glucovance*)	1.25/250 mg initially if previously untreated; 2.5/500 mg or 5/500 mg bid with meals; maximum 20/2000/d	T: 1.25/250, 2.5/500, 5/500	Starting dose should not exceed the total daily dose of either drug; see also individual drugs
Rosiglitizone and metformin (*Avandamet*)	4/1000–8/2000 in 2 divided doses	T: 1/500, 2/500, 4/500, 2/1000, 4/1000	Avoid in patients > 80 yr, Cr > 1.5 in men, Cr > 1.4 in women; see individual drugs (L, K)

Table 30. Insulin Preparations			
Preparations	Onset	Peak	Duration
Insulin lispro (*Humalog*)	15 min	0.5–1.5 h	6–8 h
Insulin (eg, *Humulin, Novolin*)*			
Regular	0.5–1 h	2–3 h	8–12 h
NPH	1–1.5 h	4–12 h	24 h
Insulin aspart (*NovoLog*)	30 min	1–3 h	3–5 h
Long-acting (*Ultralente*)	4–8 h	16–18 h	> 36 h
Insulin glargine (*Lantus*)**	1–2 h	—	24 h
Insulin, zinc (*Lente*)	1–2.5 h	8–12 h	18–24 h
Isophane insulin & regular insulin inj. (*Novolin 70/30*)	0.5 h	2–12 h	24 h

* Also available as mixtures of NPH and regular in 50:50 proportions.
** To convert from NPH dosing, give same number of units once a day. For patients taking NPH bid, decrease the total daily units by 20%, and titrate on basis of response.

Monitoring (ADA)
- Weight, BP, and foot examination, including monofilament, palpation, and inspection, each visit
- HbA_{1c} twice/yr in patients with stable glycemic control; quarterly, if poor control
- Annual comprehensive dilated eye and visual examinations by an ophthalmologist or optometrist who is experienced in management of diabetic retinopathy
- Lipid profiles every 1–2 yr depending on whether values are in normal range
- Annual (unless microalbuminuria has previously been demonstrated) test for microalbuminuria by measuring albumin-to-creatinine ratio in a random spot collection

DEFINITION
An event that results in a person's inadvertently coming to rest on the ground or lower level with or without loss of consciousness or injury. Excludes falls from major intrinsic event (seizure, stroke, syncope) or overwhelming environmental hazard.

ETIOLOGY
Typically multifactorial. Composed of intrinsic (eg, poor balance, weakness, chronic illness, visual or cognitive impairment), extrinsic (eg, polypharmacy), and environmental (eg, poor lighting, no safety equipment, loose carpets) factors. Commonly a nonspecific sign for one of many acute illnesses in older persons.

EVALUATION
Exclude acute illness or underlying systemic or metabolic process (eg, infection, electrolyte imbalance as indicated by history, examination, and laboratory studies). See **Figure 3** for recommended assessment and management. See also p 116.

- Laboratory tests for persons at risk: CBC, serum electrolytes, BUN, Cr, glucose, B_{12}, thyroid function
- Bone densitometry in women with additional risk factors for osteoporotic fracture (see p 116)
- Imaging: neuroimaging if head injury or new, focal neurologic findings on examination or if a CNS process is suspected.
- Ambulatory cardiac monitoring rarely helpful.
- Arrhythmic evaluation only if clinical evidence of this diagnosis (eg, hx of cardiac events or abnormal ECG)

History
- Circumstances of fall (eg, activity at time of fall, location, time)
- Associated symptoms (eg, lightheadedness, vertigo, syncope, weakness, confusion, palpitations)
- Relevant comorbid conditions (eg, prior stroke, parkinsonism, cardiac disease, seizure disorder, depression, anxiety, anemia, sensory deficit, glaucoma, cataracts, osteoporosis, cognitive impairment)
- Previous falls
- Medication review, including OTC medications and alcohol use; note recent changes in medications; note drugs that have hypotensive or psychoactive effects (see page 61)

Physical
Look for:
- Vital signs: postural pulse and BP changes, fever, hypothermia
- Head and neck: visual impairment (especially poor acuity, reduced contrast sensitivity, decreased visual fields, cataracts), motion-induced imbalance (Dix-Hallpike test), bruit, nystagmus
- Musculoskeletal: arthritic changes, motion or joint limitations (especially lower extremity joint function), postural instability, skeletal deformities, podiatric problems

Figure 3. Assessment and Management of Falls

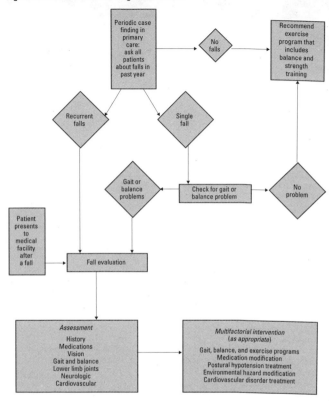

Sources: Adapted from American Geriatrics Society, British Geriatrics Society, and American Academy of Orthopaedic Surgeons Panel on Falls Prevention. Guideline for the prevention of falls in older persons. *J Amer Geriatr Soc.* 2001; 49(5):666, and Tinetti M. Preventing falls in elderly persons. *N Engl J Med* 2003;348(1):42–49.

- Neurologic: slower reflexes, altered proprioception, altered mental status, focal deficits, peripheral neuropathy, gait or balance disorders, muscle weakness (especially leg), instability, tremor, rigidity
- Cardiovascular: heart arrhythmias, cardiac valve dysfunction
- Other: fever; hypothermia

Functional Assessment
• Functional gait: observe patient rising from chair, walking (stride, length, velocity, symmetry), turning, sitting (Timed Get Up and Go test; see also POMA, p 187)
• Balance: Side-by-side, semi-tandem, and full tandem stance; Functional Reach test (see also POMA, p 187)
• Mobility: observe the patient's use of assistive device (cane, walker, or personal assistance), extent of ambulation, restraint use, footwear evaluation
Ask about person's ability to complete activities of daily living: bathing, dressing, transferring, continence.

Medications Associated with Increased Fall Risk
• Neuroleptics (especially phenothiazines)
• Sedatives, hypnotics (including benzodiazepines)
• Antidepressants (including MAOIs, SSRIs, TCAs)
• Antiarrhythmics (Class 1A)
• Anticonvulsants

PREVENTION
Goal is to minimize risk of falling without compromising mobility and functional independence.
• Fall risk assessment should be part of every routine primary health care visit (at least annually). Risk of falling significantly increases as number of risk factors increases.
• Assess for risk factors using a multidisciplinary approach, if appropriate, including medical and occupational therapy.
  - Diagnose and treat underlying cause.
• Target interventions to risk factors (see **Table 31**). Correction of postural hypotension, review and elimination or dose reduction of medications, and interventions to improve balance, transfers, and gait are priority.
• Choose fall prevention programs that include more than one intervention. A structured, interdisciplinary approach should be used.
  - Establish tailored exercise programs targeted at older people without balance or gait difficulties that includes balance and strength training.
  - Tai Chi classes should be offered to older people living in the community.
  - Counsel older patients or family members on multifactorial nature of most falls, specific risk factors, and measures to reduce the risk of falling, including exercise, safety-related skills and behaviors, and environmental hazard reduction.
  - Offer hip protectors to all residents of nursing homes and others at high risk—available via www.hipprotector.com or www.hipsaver.com.
• Focus on most common risk factors: Muscle weakness, history of falls, gait deficit, balance deficit, use of assistive devices, visual deficit, arthritis, impaired ADLs, depression, cognitive impairment, age > 80 yr.

Table 31. Preventing Falls: Selected Risk Factors and Suggested Interventions

Factors	Suggested Interventions
Medication-related factors	
Use of benzodiazepines, sedative-hypnotics, or antipsychotic	Consider agents with less risk for falls (eg, atypical antipsychotics such as olanzapine, risperidone, or quetiapine)
	Taper and D/C medications, as possible
	Address sleep problems with nonpharmacologic interventions (see p 166)
	Educate regarding appropriate use of medications and monitoring for side effects
Recent change in dose *or* number of prescriptions medications *or* use of ≥ 4 prescription medications *or* use of other medications associated with fall risk	Review medication profile and modify, as possible
	Monitor response to medications and to dose changes
Mobility-related factors	
Presence of environmental hazards (eg, improper bed height, cluttered walking surfaces, lack of railings, poor lighting)	Improve lighting, especially at night
	Remove floor barriers (eg, loose carpeting)
	Replace existing furniture with safer furniture (eg, correct height, more stable)
	Install support structures (eg, railings, grab bars)
	Use nonslip bathmats
Impaired gait, balance, or transfer skills	Refer to PT for comprehensive evaluation and rehabilitation
	Gait training
	Balance or strengthening exercises
	Provide training in transfer skills
	Prescribe appropriate assistive devices
	Recommend protective hip padding
	Environmental changes (eg, grab bars, raised toilet seats)
	Recommend appropriate footwear
Impaired leg or arm strength or range of motion, or proprioception	Strengthening exercises (eg, use of resistive rubber bands, putty)
	Resistance training 2–3 times/wk to 10 repetitions with full range of motion, then increase resistance
	Tai Chi
	Physical therapy
Medical factors	
Parkinson's disease, osteoarthritis, depressive symptoms, impaired cognition, other conditions associated with increased falls	Optimize medical therapy
	Monitor for disease progression and impact on mobility and impairments
	Determine need for assistive devices
Postural hypotension: drop in SBP ≥ 20 mm Hg (or ≥ 20%) with or without symptoms, either immediately or within 2 min of standing	Review medications potentially contributing and adjust dosing or switch to less hypotensive agents; avoid vasodilators and diuretics if possible
	Educate on activities to decrease effect (eg, slow rising, ankle pumps, hand clenching, elevation of head of bed) and slow rising from recumbent or seated position
	Prescribe pressure stockings (eg, Jobst)
	Liberalize salt intake
	Caffeinated coffee (1 cup) or caffeine 100 mg with meals for postprandial hypotension
	Consider medication to increase pressure (if hypertension, heart failure, and hypokalemia not serious):
	-fludrocortisone (*Florinef*) 0.1 mg qd–tid [T: 0.1]
	-midodrine (*ProAmatine*) 2.5–5 mg tid [T: 2.5, 5]

GASTROINTESTINAL DISEASES

DYSPHAGIA
See p 128.

GASTROESOPHAGEAL REFLUX DISEASE (GERD)

Definition
The retrograde movement of the gastric contents in the esophagus due to incompetent lower esophageal sphincter, transient relaxations of the sphincter, or compromise of other antireflux mechanisms.

Evaluation and Assessment
Empiric treatment is appropriate when hx is typical for uncomplicated GERD.
• Endoscopy (if symptoms persist despite initial management, atypical presentation, or longstanding symptoms)
• 24-h pH monitoring

Symptoms Suggesting Complicated GERD and Need For Evaluation
• Dysphagia
• Bleeding
• Weight loss
• Choking (acid causing cough, SOB, or hoarseness)
• Chest pain

Management
Nonpharmacologic:
• Antacids
• Avoid alcohol and fatty foods
• Avoid lying down 3 h after eating
• Avoid tight-fitting clothes
• Change diet (avoid pepper, spearmint, chocolate, spicy or acidic foods)
• Drink 6–8 oz water with all medications
• Elevate head of the bed (6–8 in)
• Lose weight (if overweight)
• Stop drugs that may promote reflux
• Stop smoking
• Consider surgery

Pharmacologic:

Table 32. Pharmacologic Management of GERD		
Drug	**Initial Oral Dosage**	**Formulations (Excretion)**
Proton-Pump Inhibitors		
Esomeprazole (*Nexium*)	20 mg qd × 4 wk	C: ER 20, 40 (L)
Lansoprazole (*Prevacid*)	15 mg qd × 8 wk	C: ER 15, 30; granules for susp: 15, 30/packet (L)
Omeprazole (*Prilosec*)	20 mg qd × 4–8 wk	C: ER 10, 20,* 40 (L)
Pantoprazole (*Protonix*)	40 mg qd × 8 wk	T: enteric-coated, 20, 40; Inj (L)
Rabeprazole (*Aciphex*)	20 mg qd × 4–8 wk; 20 mg qd maintenance, if needed	T: enteric-coated ER 20 (L)
H₂ Antagonists (for less severe GERD)		
Cimetidine (*Tagamet*)	400 or 800 mg bid	S: 200 mg/20 mL, 300 mg/5 mL with alcohol 2.8%; T: 100, 200,* 300, 400, 800; Inj (K, L)

(continues)

Table 32. Pharmacologic Management of GERD (cont.)		
Drug	**Initial Oral Dosage**	**Formulations (Excretion)**
Famotidine (*Pepcid*)	20 mg bid × 6 wk	S: oral sus 40 mg/5 mL; T: film-coated 10,* 20, 40, oral disintegrating 20, 40; C (gel): 10*; ChT: 10*; Inj (K)
Nizatidine (*Axid*)	150 mg bid	C: 150, 300; T: 75 (K)
Ranitidine (*Zantac*)	150 mg bid	Pk: gran, effervescent (EFFERdose) 150 mg; S: syr 15 mg/mL; T: 75,* 150, 300; T: effervescent (EFFERdose) 150; Inj (K, F)
Mucosal Protective Agent		
Sucralfate (*Carafate*)	1 g qid, 1h ac and hs	S: oral sus 1 g/10 mL; T: 1 g (F, K)
Prokinetic Agents		
Bethanechol (*Urecholine*)	25 mg qid	T: 5, 10, 25, 50 (unknown)
Metoclopramide† (*Reglan*)	5 mg qid, ac, and hs	S: syr, sugar-free 5 mg/5 mL, conc 10 mg/mL; T: 5, 10; Inj (K, F)

* OTC strength.
† Risk of extrapyramidal symptoms high in persons aged > 65 yr.
Source: Data from DeVault KR, Castell DO. Updated guidelines for the diagnosis and treatment of gastroesophageal reflux disease. *Am J Gastroenterol.* 1999;94:1430–1442.

PEPTIC ULCER DISEASE
Causes
Helicobacter pylori is the major cause. NSAIDs are the second most common cause.

Diagnosis of *H pylori*
- Endoscopic examination
- Serology
- Urea breath test

Initial Treatment Options
- Empiric anti-ulcer treatment for 6 wk
- Definitive diagnostic evaluation by endoscopy
- Noninvasive testing for *H pylori* and treatment with antibiotics for (+) patients (see **Table 33** for regimens)
- Review patient's chronic medications for drug interactions before selecting regimen; many potential drug interactions and adverse drug reactions.

Table 33. FDA-Approved Treatments for *H. pylori*–Induced Ulcerations (all oral routes)
Lansoprazole 30 mg bid + amoxicillin 1 g bid + clarithromycin 500 mg tid × 10 (or 14) d
or Omeprazole 20 mg bid + clarithromycin 500 mg bid + amoxicillin 1 g bid × 10 d
or Lansoprazole 30 mg bid + clarithromycin 500 mg bid + amoxicillin 1 g bid × 10 d (*Prevpac*)
or Omeprazole 40 mg qd + clarithromycin 500 mg tid × 2 wk, then omeprazole 20 mg qd × 2 wk
or Lansoprazole 30 mg tid + amoxicillin 1 g bid × 2 wk (only for person allergic or intolerant to clarithromycin)

or Ranitidine bismuth citrate (RBC) 400 mg bid + clarithromycin 500 mg tid × 2 wk, then RBC 400 mg bid × 2 wk

or RBC 400 mg bid + clarithromycin 500 mg bid × 2 wk, then RBC 400 mg bid × 2 wk

or Bismuth subsalicylate (*Pepto-Bismol*) 525 mg qid (pc and hs) + metronidazole 250 mg qid + tetracycline 500 mg qid × 2 wk (*Helidac*) + H$_2$ receptor antagonist therapy as directed × 4 wk

Source: www.cdc.gov/ulcer/md.htm.
For additional, non-FDA approved regimens, see Howden CW, Hunt RH. Guidelines for the management of *Helicobacter pylori* infection. *Am J Gastroenterol* 1998;93:2330–2338, or www.acg.gi.org.

Medications
Bismuth subsalicylate (*Pepto-Bismol*) [T: 324; ChT: 262; S: sus 262 mg/15 mL, 525 mg/15 mL]
Antibiotics: (for complete information, see **Table 46**)
Amoxicillin (*Amoxil*) [C: 250, 500; ChT: 125, 250; S: oral sus 125 mg/5 mL, 250 mg/5 mL]
Clarithromycin (*Biaxin*) [T: film-coated 250, 500; S: oral sus 125 mg/5 mL, 250 mg/5 mL]
Metronidazole (*Flagyl*) [T: 250, 500, 750; C: 375]
Tetracycline (*Achromycin, Sumycin*) [T: 250, 500; S: oral sus 125 mg/5 mL]
Proton-Pump Inhibitors: See **Table 32**.

STRESS-ULCER PREVENTION IN HOSPITALIZED OLDER PERSONS
Risk Factors (in order of prevalence in older persons)
• Hx of GI ulceration or bleed in the past year
• Sepsis
• Multiple organ failure
• Hypotension
• Respiratory failure requiring mechanical ventilation > 48 h
• Renal failure
• Major trauma, shock, or head injury
• Coagulopathy (platelets < 50,000/μL, INR > 1.5, or PTT > 2 × control)
• Burns over > 25% of body surface area
• Hepatic failure
• Intracranial hypertension
• Spinal cord injury
• Tetraplegia
Prophylaxis
• H$_2$ antagonists (see **Table 32**)
• Proton-pump inhibitors (see **Table 32**)
• Sucralfate (see **Table 32**)
• Antacids
• Enteral feedings
Discontinue H$_2$ antagonists, proton-pump inhibitors, and other treatments for stress ulcer prevention before transfer or discharge.

Key points
- Prophylaxis has not been shown to reduce mortality
- No one regimen has shown superior efficacy
- Choice of regimen depends on access to and function of GI tract and presence of nasogastric suction

CONSTIPATION
Definition
Infrequent, incomplete, or painful evacuation of feces.

Drugs That Constipate
- Analgesics—opiates
- Antacids with aluminum or calcium
- Anticholinergic drugs
- Antidepressants, lithium
- Antihypertensives
- Antipsychotics
- Barium sulfate
- Bismuth
- Calcium channel blockers
- Diuretics
- Iron

Conditions That Constipate
- Colon tumor or mechanical obstruction
- Dehydration
- Depression
- Diabetes mellitus
- Hypercalcemia
- Hypokalemia
- Hypothyroidism
- Immobility
- Low intake of fiber
- Panhypopituitarism
- Parkinson's disease
- Spinal cord injury
- Stroke
- Uremia

Management of Chronic Constipation
Step 1. Stop all constipating medications, when possible.
Step 2. Increase dietary bran to 6–25 g/d, increase fluid intake to ≥ 1500 mL/d, and increase physical activity; or add bran supplements, provided fluid intake is ≥ 1500 mL/d.
Step 3. Add 70% sorbitol solution (15–30 mL qd or bid, max 150 mL/d).
Step 4. Add stimulant laxative (eg, senna, bisacodyl), 2–3 times/wk. (Alternative: Saline laxative, but avoid in renal insufficiency.)
Step 5. Use tap water enema or saline enema 2 times/wk.
Step 6. Use oil-retention enema for refractory constipation.

Table 34. Medications That May Relieve Constipation			
Medication	Onset of Action	Starting Dosage	Site and Mechanism of Action
Bisacodyl tablet (*Dulcolax*)	6–10 h	5–15 mg × 1	Colon; increases peristalsis
Bisacodyl suppository (*Dulcolax*)	0.25–1 h	10 mg × 1	Colon; increases peristalsis
Docusate (*Colace*)	24–72 h	100 mg qd–qid	Small and large intestine; detergent activity; facilitates admixture of fat and water to soften stool

Table 34. Medications That May Relieve Constipation (cont.)			
Medication	**Onset of Action**	**Starting Dosage**	**Site and Mechanism of Action**
Lactulose (*Cephulac*)*	24–48 h	15–30 mL qd–bid	Colon; osmotic effect
Magnesium citrate (*Citroma*)	0.5–3 h	120–240 mL × 1	Small and large intestine; attracts, retains water in intestinal lumen
Magnesium hydroxide (*Milk of Magnesia*)	30 min–3 h	30 mL qd–bid	Osmotic effect and increased peristalsis in colon
Methylcellulose psyllium (*Metamucil*)	12–24 h (up to 72 h)	1–2 rounded tsp or packets qd–tid with water or juice	Small and large intestine; holds water in stool; mechanical distention
Polyethylene glycol (*MiraLax*)*	48–96 h	17 g pwd qd (~1 tablespoon) dissolved in 8 oz water	GI tract; osmotic effect
Sodium phosphate/ biphosphate emollient enema (*Fleet*)	2–15 min	1 4.5-oz enema × 1, repeat prn	Colon
Senna (*Senoket*)	6–10 h	2 tabs or 1 tsp qhs	Colon; direct action on intestine; stimulates myenteric plexus; alters water and electrolyte secretion
Sorbitol 70%	24–48 h	15–30 mL qd–bid	Colon; delivers osmotically active molecules to colon

* By prescription only.

NAUSEA AND VOMITING
Causes
- CNS disorders (eg, motion sickness, intracranial lesions)
- Drugs (eg, chemotherapy, NSAIDs, narcotic analgesics, antibiotics, digoxin)
- GI disorders (eg, mechanical obstruction; inflammation of stomach, intestine, or gallbladder; pseudo-obstruction, motility disorders, dyspepsia, diabetic gastroparesis)
- Infections (eg, viral or bacterial gastroenteritis, hepatitis, otitis, meningitis)
- Metabolic conditions (eg, uremia, acidosis, hyperparathyroidism, adrenal insufficiency)
- Psychiatric disorders

Evaluation
- If patient is not seriously ill or dehydrated, can probably wait 24–48 h to see if symptoms resolve spontaneously.
- If patient is seriously ill, dehydrated, or has other signs of acute illness, hospitalize for further evaluation.
- If symptoms persist, evaluate according to suspected causes.

Pharmacologic Management

Drugs that are useful in the management of nausea and vomiting are listed in **Table 35**.

Table 35. Selected Antiemetics		
Drug	**Formulations**	**Dosages (Metabolism)**
Dimenhydrinate* (*Dramamine*)	Inj; S: 12.5 mg/4 mL, 16.62 mg/ 5 mL; T: 50; ChT: 50	Oral, IM IV; 50–100 mg q 4–6 h, not to exceed 400 mg/d (L)
Meclizine* (*Antivert*)	C: 25, 30; T: 12.5, 25, 50; ChT: 25; T: film-coated 25	Motion sickness: 12.5–25 mg 1 h before travel, repeat dose q 12–24 h if needed; doses up to 50 mg may be needed; vertigo: 25–100 mg/d in divided doses (L)
Metoclopramide (*Reglan*)	Inj; S: oral conc 10 mg/mL, syr, sugar-free, 5 mg/5 mL; T: 5, 10	Chemotherapy-induced emesis, IV: 1–2 mg/kg 30 min before chemotherapy and q 2–4 to q 4–6 h; postoperative nausea and vomiting: IM 5–10 mg near the end of surgery (K)
Prochlorperazine (*Compazine*)	C: ER: 10, 15, 30; Inj; Sp: 2.5, 5, 25; S: syr 5 mg/5 mL; T: 5, 10, 25	Oral or IM: 5–10 mg 3–4 times/d, usual maximum, 40 mg/d; IV: 2.5–10 mg; maximum 10 mg/dose or 40 mg/d; may repeat dose q 3–4 h as needed; rectal: 25 mg bid (L)

* Available OTC.
Note: All have potential CNS toxicity.

DIARRHEA
Causes
• Drugs (eg, antibiotics [see **Table 46**], laxatives, colchicine)
• Fecal impaction
• GI disorders (eg, irritable bowel syndrome, malabsorption, inflammatory bowel disease)
• Infections (eg, viral, bacterial, parasitic)
• Lactose intolerance

Evaluation
• If patient is not seriously ill or dehydrated and there is no blood in the stool, can probably wait 48 h to see if symptoms resolve spontaneously.
• If patient is seriously ill, dehydrated, or has other signs of acute illness, hospitalize for further evaluation.
• If diarrhea persists, evaluate on the basis of the most likely causes.

Pharmacologic Management

Drugs that are useful in the management of diarrhea are listed in **Table 36**.

Table 36. Antidiarrheals		
Drug	**Dosage (Metabolism)**	**Formulations**
√ Attapulgite* (*Kaopectate*)	1200–1500 mg after each loose bowel movement or q 2 h; 15–30 mL up to 9 × /d, up to 9000 mg/24 h (not absorbed)	S: oral conc 600, 750 mg/ 15 mL; T: 750; ChT: 300, 600
√ Bismuth subsalicylate* (*Pepto-Bismol*)	2 tablets or 30 mL q 30 min to 1 h as needed up to 8 doses/ 24 h	S: 262 mg/15 mL, 525 mg/ 15 mL; T: 324; ChT: 262
Diphenoxylate with atropine (*Lomotil*)†	15–20 mg/d of diphenoxylate in 3–4 divided doses; maintenance 5–15 mg/d in 2–3 divided doses (L)	S: oral, diphenoxylate hydrochloride 2.5 mg + atropine sulfate 0.025 mg/5 mL; T: diphenoxylate hydrochloride 2.5 mg and atropine sulfate 0.025 mg
√ Loperamide* (*Imodium A-D*)	Initial: 4 mg (2 capsules), followed by 2 mg after each loose stool, up to 16 mg/d (8 capsules) (L)	Caplet, 2; C: 2; T: 2; S: oral, 1 mg/5 mL

√ = preferred for treating older persons.
* Available OTC.
† Anticholinergic, potentially CNS toxic.

ANTIBIOTIC-ASSOCIATED DIARRHEA
(Antibiotic-associated pseudomembranous colitis, or AAPMC)

Definition
A specific form of *Clostridium difficile* pseudomembranous colitis

Risk Factors
Almost any oral or parenteral antibiotic and several antineoplastic agents, including cyclophosphamide, doxorubicin, fluorouracil, methotrexate.

Presentation
- Abdominal pain, cramping
- Dehydration
- Diarrhea (can be bloody)
- Fecal leukocytes
- Fever (100–105°F)
- Hypoalbuminemia
- Hypovolemia
- Leukocytosis

Symptoms appear a few days after starting to 10 wk after discontinuing the offending agent.

Diagnosis
- Isolation of *C difficile* or its toxin from symptomatic patient. Three negative stools are needed to exclude diagnosis.
- Lower endoscopy; however, lesions may be scattered.

Treatment
- Discontinue offending agent if possible.
- Metronidazole (*Flagyl*) 250 mg po qid or 500 mg po tid × 10 d or vancomycin 125–500 mg po qid × 10 d.
- Treat diarrhea with cholestyramine resin (eg, *Questran*) 4 g 1–6 ×/d to adsorb toxin.
- Avoid opiates or other agents that will slow GI motility.

Recurrence
Relapse seen in 10% to 20% of patients 1–4 wk after treatment (spore-producing organism). Re-treat with same regimen or use alternative.

DEFINITION
The most common sensory impairment in old age. To quantify hearing ability, the necessary intensity (decibel = dB) and frequency (Hertz) of the perceived pure-tone signal must be described.

EVALUATION
Screening
- Note problems during conversation
- Ask about hearing dysfunction
- Use a standardized questionnaire (see p 186)
- Test with handheld audioscope

- Use whisper test—stand behind patient 2 ft from ear, cover untested ear, fully exhale, whisper an easily answered question
- Refer patients who screen positive for audiologic evaluation

Audiometry
- Documents the dB loss across frequencies
- Determines the pattern of loss (see Classification, below)

- Determines if loss is unilateral or bilateral **Note:** If speech discrimination is less than 50%, results with hearing aids may be poor

Aggravating Factors
- Sensorineural loss—medication ototoxicity (eg, aminoglycosides, loop diuretics, cisplatin), cerumen impaction (see p 72)
- Conductive loss—cerumen impaction, external otitis

CLASSIFICATION
Sensorineural Hearing Loss
Due to cochlear or retrocochlear pathology; both air and bone conduction thresholds are increased; causes: aging, eighth nerve damage from syphilis, viral meningitis, trauma, vascular events to eighth nerve or cortical tracts, acoustic neuroma, Ménière's disease.

Conductive Hearing Loss
Occurs when sound transmission to inner ear is impaired; bone conduction better than air conduction; causes include: external or middle ear disorders, including otosclerosis; rheumatoid arthritis; Paget's disease.

Central Auditory Processing Disorder
Loss of speech discrimination in excess of that from loss in hearing sensitivity; involves the CNS; occurs in dementia and infrequently with presbycusis.

Presbycusis (Old-Age Hearing Loss, a Subtype of Sensorineural Loss):
- Mainly high-frequency loss
- Impaired speech discrimination

- Recruitment (an increase in sensation of loudness)
- Both bone and air conduction affected

MANAGEMENT
Remove Ear Wax

Fill ear canal with 5–10 gtt water and cover with cotton bid × 4 d or more. Liquid must stay in contact with ear for at least 15 min. Hearing may worsen as cerumen expands. Water is as effective as commercial preparations (eg, *Debrox, Cerumenex, Colace*). Use of any of the commercial preparations for more than 4 d may cause ear irritation.

Table 37. Effects and Rehabilitation of Hearing Loss, by Level of Loss		
Level of Loss	**Difficulty Understanding**	**Need for Hearing Aid**
0–24 dB	None	None
25–40 dB (mild)	Normal speech	In specific situations
41–55 dB (moderate)	Loud speech	Frequent
56–80 dB (severe)	Anything but amplified speech	For all communication
81 dB or more (profound)	Even amplified speech	Plus speech reading, aural rehabilitation, sign language, or cochlear implants

Source: Data in part from *A Report on Hearing Aids: User Perspectives and Concerns.* Washington, DC: American Association of Retired Persons; 1993:2.

Hearing Devices

Hearing Aids: Appropriate for most hearing-impaired persons; enhance select frequencies; should be individualized for each ear. Amplification in both ears (binaural) achieves best speech understanding; unilateral aid may be appropriate if asymmetrical speech discrimination, if hearing aid care is challenging, or because of cost.

Assistive Listening Devices: Microphone placed close to sound source transmits to headphones or earpiece. Transmission is by wire or wireless (FM or infrared); these systems increase signal-to-noise ratio, which is useful for persons with central auditory processing disorder.

Telephone Device for the Deaf (TDD): Receiver is a keyboard that allows the hearing-impaired person to respond.

Cochlear Implants: Bypass the middle ear, directly innervate auditory nerve. Reserved for severe and profound hearing loss. Results after age 65 comparable to younger persons. Failure rate < 1%, but patient selection important.

Tips for Communication with Hearing-Impaired Persons

- Stand 2–3 ft away
- Have the person's attention
- Have the person seated in front of a wall, which will help reflect sound
- Use lower-pitched voice
- Speak slowly and distinctly; don't shout
- Rephrase rather than repeat
- Pause at the end of phrases or ideas

ANEMIA
Evaluation
- Some decrease in Hb with age is normal.
- Evaluate persons > 65 when Hb < 13.
- Evaluate if Hb falls > 1 g/dL in 1 yr.
- Physical examination and laboratory tests to look for kidney or liver disease.
- Evaluate GI and GU source if iron deficient.
- Check WBC and peripheral blood smear, and pursue suspected causes as appropriate.
- Combined deficiencies are common in older people; reasonable to check B_{12}, folate, and iron in all cases
- Check reticulocyte count and reticulocyte index.
  - Reticulocyte count/index high: adequate response, suspect blood loss or RBC destruction
  - Reticulocyte count/index normal or low, check MCV
    ○ MCV >100 μm^3/cell: see **Figure 4**
    ○ MCV <100 μm^3/cell: see **Figure 5**

Diagnosis: Common Anemias of Later Life
Iron deficiency anemia: usual laboratory values (Fe, TIBC, ferritin) less reliable in presence of other conditions (see **Figure 5**).
Chronic disease anemia:
- Most common causes in elderly people are:
  - acute and chronic infection
  - chronic inflammation
  - malignancy
  - protein calorie malnutrition
  - unidentified chronic disease
- Laboratory tests: usually low iron, low or normal TIBC, high ferritin, low soluble transferrin receptor
- Type determines treatability:
  - "rheumatoid arthritis type" responds to erythropoietin at usual doses (see **Table 38**)
  - "cancer type" may respond to erythropoietin at high doses (see **Table 38**)
- Restoring Hb to higher levels improves quality of life, function, and possibly survival.
Anemia of renal insufficiency:
- Caused by decreased erythropoietin production
- Restoring Hb levels increases survival, quality of life, and cognitive function, and decreases hospitalization, LVH, and HF. Treatment is erythropoietin (see **Table 38**).
Anemia of B_{12} and folate deficiency:
- Laboratory tests: anemia or pancytopenia, macrocytosis
- B_{12} deficiency definite at levels < 100 pg/mL, possible at levels of 100–300; check MMA or give trial of B_{12} replacement (see **Figure 5**)
- Treatment: see **Table 38**

Figure 4. Evaluation of Hypoproliferative Anemia with Elevated MCV

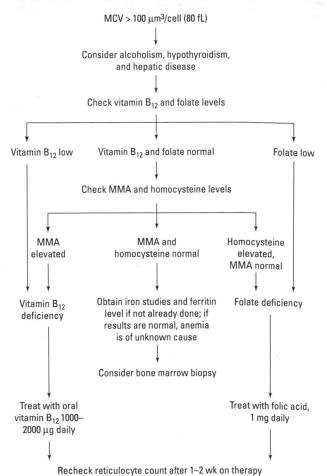

MCV > 100 μm³/cell (80 fL)

↓

Consider alcoholism, hypothyroidism, and hepatic disease

↓

Check vitamin B₁₂ and folate levels

Vitamin B₁₂ low — Vitamin B₁₂ and folate normal — Folate low

Check MMA and homocysteine levels

MMA elevated — MMA and homocysteine normal — Homocysteine elevated, MMA normal

Vitamin B₁₂ deficiency — Obtain iron studies and ferritin level if not already done; if results are normal, anemia is of unknown cause — Folate deficiency

Consider bone marrow biopsy

Treat with oral vitamin B₁₂ 1000–2000 μg daily — Treat with folic acid, 1 mg daily

Recheck reticulocyte count after 1–2 wk on therapy

Source: Balducci L. Epidemiology of anemia in the elderly: Information on diagnostic evaluation. *J Amer Geriatr Soc* 2003; 51(3 Suppl):S2–9. Reprinted with permission.

Figure 5. Evaluation of Hypoproliferative Anemia with Normal or Low MCV

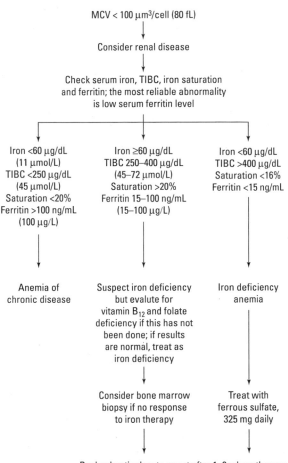

MCV < 100 μm³/cell (80 fL)

↓

Consider renal disease

↓

Check serum iron, TIBC, iron saturation and ferritin; the most reliable abnormality is low serum ferritin level

Iron <60 μg/dL (11 μmol/L) TIBC <250 μg/dL (45 μmol/L) Saturation <20% Ferritin >100 ng/mL (100 μg/L)	Iron ≥60 μg/dL TIBC 250–400 μg/dL (45–72 μmol/L) Saturation >20% Ferritin 15–100 ng/mL (15–100 μg/L)	Iron <60 μg/dL TIBC >400 μg/dL Saturation <16% Ferritin <15 ng/mL
Anemia of chronic disease	Suspect iron deficiency but evaluate for vitamin B₁₂ and folate deficiency if this has not been done; if results are normal, treat as iron deficiency	Iron deficiency anemia
	Consider bone marrow biopsy if no response to iron therapy	Treat with ferrous sulfate, 325 mg daily

Recheck reticulocyte count after 1–2 wk on therapy

Source: Balducci L. Epidemiology of anemia in the elderly: Information on diagnostic evaluation. *J Amer Geriatr Soc* 2003; 51(3 Suppl):S2–9. Reprinted with permission.

Anemia of unknown cause:
- Prevalence: 17% of all anemias after age 65
- May be age-related decline in hematopoietic reserve, low erythropoietin, and/or poor response to endogenous erythropoietin

Pancytopenia:
- Unless due to B_{12} deficiency, bone marrow aspirate is indicated
- Causes include cancer, fibrosis, myelodysplasia
- Aplastic anemia increases in prevalence with age; 50% respond to antithymocyte globulin and cyclosporine

Table 38. Treatment of Anemias Associated with Deficiency		
Treatment	**Formulation and Dosage**	**Comments**
Iron	Ferrous sulfate 325 mg po qd	Higher doses cause more GI side effects
	Ferrous polysaccharide 50 mg po qd	Fewer GI side effects
	Iron dextran	For severe deficiency or poor absorption
	Dose (mL) = 0.0442 (desired Hb − observed Hb) × LBW (kg) + (0.26 × LBW). For LBW, see p X. Administer test dose at 0.5 mL IM or IV sol (5 gtt/min). Wait 30–45 min. If tolerated, complete dose by slow IM injection ≤ 50 mg/min. By IV, dilute dose in 500 mL normal saline (45–60 mL/min).	
B_{12}	1000 μg IM every wk × 5, then 1000 μg IM every mo or 1000 μg po qd	Monitor K^+ in first wk of treatment
Folate	1 mg po qd	
Erythropoietin	Epogen alfa (*Epogen*) usual dose 50–150 U/kg SC every wk	Monitor BP, adjust dose based on response; Medicare pays for use in renal failure and in anemia due to chemotherapy
	Darbepoietin alfa (*Aranesp*) 0.45 μg/kg every wk	See full prescribing information for titration

CANCER
Many older persons receive long-term drug therapy for cancers of the breast and prostate.

Breast Cancer
Prevention: Also see **Table 62**. Tamoxifen 20 mg po qd reduces breast cancer risk by 49% in women at high risk. For risk assessment see prevention section of www.cancer.gov/cancerinfo/prevention_genetics_causes/breast

Monitoring:
- History, physical
- LFTs, calcium every 4–6 mo for 5 yr, then yearly
- Annual mammography, pelvic, and FOBT

Oral Hormone Adjuvant Therapy: Postmenopausal women with estrogen receptor (ER) or progesterone receptor (PR) positive tumors at high risk for recurrence (tumors greater than 1 cm, or positive nodes) should be treated with oral adjuvant therapy for 5 yr, even when treated with chemotherapy. See **Table 39**.

Adjuvant Chemotherapy: Reduces recurrence risk for receptor-negative tumors. There is an additional 5% to 10% reduction in recurrence in ER- or PR-positive tumors treated with both tamoxifen and chemotherapy.

Therapy for Metastatic Bone Disease: Pamidronate or zoledronic acid reduces morbidity and delays time to onset of bone symptoms. Consult oncology.

Table 39. Oral Agents for Breast Cancer Treatment				
Class, Agent	Dosage	Formulations	Monitoring	Comments
Anti-estrogen Drugs				
Fulvestrant (*Faslodex*)	250 mg IM 1/mo in 1 or 2 injections	Inj	Blood chemistry, lipids	Has potent CYP3A4 inhibitors; GI reactions, anesthesia, pain (back, pelvic, headache), hot flushes
Tamoxifen* (*Nolvadex*)	20 mg po qd	T: 10, 20	Annual eye exam; endometrial cancer screening	Drug interactions: erythromycin, calcium channel blockers; ↑ risk of thrombosis
Toremifene (*Fareston*)	60 mg po qd	T: 60	CBC, Ca, LFTs, BUN, Cr	Drug interactions with CYP3A4–6 inhibitors and inducers (see **Table 7**); ↑ warfarin effect
Aromatase Inhibitors				
Exemestane (*Aromasin*)	25 mg po qd	T: 25	Periodic WBC with differential, lipids, serum chemistry profile	Second- or third-line therapy after tamoxifen failure
Letrozole† (*Femara*)	2.5 mg po qd	T: 2.5	Periodic CBC, LFTs, TSH	First-line therapy for hormone-responsive metastatic disease or tamoxifen failure
Anastrozole† (*Arimidex*)	1 mg po qd	T: 1	Periodic CBC, lipids, serum chemistry profile	Same as letrozole

*Reduce dose if CrCl < 10 mL/min.
† In head-to-head trials, these aromatase inhibitors have lower recurrence rates than tamoxifen; both are more effective than tamoxifen in advanced inoperable disease. In one large randomized trial, aromatase inhibitors were superior to tamoxifen as adjuvant therapy in postmenopausal women.

Prostate Cancer
PSA: See **Table 62**.
Histology:
• Gleason score 2–6 has low 15–20 yr morbidity and mortality; watchful waiting usually appropriate.
• Gleason score ≥ 7, higher PSA and younger age associated with higher morbidity and mortality; best treatment strategy (surgery, radiation, androgen suppression, etc) is not known.

Pharmacotherapy: Hormonal therapy is indicated in locally advanced ≥ stage III or T3 (tumor extension beyond the prostate capsule) and metastatic prostate cancer. Treatment of earlier stage disease is controversial. No luteinizing hormone-releasing hormone (LH–RH) agent is superior to others; they vary only in side-effect profile. Combining forms of androgen blockade has no advantage over monotherapy.

Table 40. Common Drugs for Prostate Cancer Therapy			
Class, Agent	**Dosage**	**Metabolism**	**Side Effects**
LH-RH agonists			
Goserelin acetate implant (*Zoladex*)	3.6 mg SC q 28 d or 10.8 mg q 3 mo	Rapid urinary and hepatic excretion, no dose adjustment in renal impairment	Side effects: hot flushes (60%), breast swelling, libido change, impotence, nausea
Leuprolide acetate (*Lupron Depot*)	7.5 mg IM q mo or 22.5 mg q 3 mo or 30 mg q 4 mo	Unknown; active metabolites for 4–12 wk, dose-dependent	Certain symptoms (obstruction, spinal cord compression, bone pain) may be exacerbated early in treatment; side effects: hot flushes (60%), edema (12%), pain (7%), nausea, vomiting, impotence, dyspnea, asthenia (all 5%), thrombosis, PE, MI (all 1%); headache as high as 32%
Triptorelin (*Trelstar Depot, Trelstar LA*)	Depot: 375 mg q 28 d IM LA: 11.25 mg q 84 d IM	Hepatic metabolism and renal excretion (42% as intact peptide)	Hot flushes, ↑ glucose, ↓ Hgb, ↓ RBC, ↑ alk phos, ALT/AST, skeletal pain, ↑ BUN
Antiandrogens			Class side effects: nausea, hot flushes, breast pain, gynecomastia, hematuria, diarrhea, liver enzyme elevations, galactorrhea
Bicalutamide (*Casodex*)	50 mg po qd [T: 50]	Metabolized in liver, excreted in urine; half-life 10 d at steady state	
Flutamide (*Eulexin*)	125 mg cap 2 po q 8 h [C: 125]	Renally excreted; half-life 5–6 h	Greatest GI toxicity in the class; severe liver dysfunction reported
Nilutamide (*Nilandron*)	300 mg for 30 d, then 150 mg po qd [T: 50]	80% protein bound; liver metabolism, renal excretion; half-life 40–60 h	Delayed light adaptation

PNEUMONIA

Presentation

Can range from subtle signs such as lethargy, anorexia, dizziness, falls, and delirium to septic shock or adult respiratory distress syndrome. Pleuritic chest pain, dyspnea, productive cough, fever, chills, or rigors are not consistently present in older patients.

Evaluation and Assessment

- Physical examination: Respiratory rate > 20 breaths/min; low BP, chest sounds may be minimal, absent, or consistent with HF; temperature: 20% will be afebrile.
- CXR: Infiltrate may not be present on initial film if the patient is dehydrated.
- Sputum Gram's stain and culture (optional per ATS guidelines)
- CBC with differential: Up to 50% of patients have a normal white blood cell count, but 95% have a left shift.
- BUN, creatinine, electrolytes, glucose
- Blood culture × 2
- Oxygenation: arterial blood gas or oximetry
- Test for *Mycobacterium tuberculosis* with acid fast bacilli strain and culture in selected patients.
- Test for *Legionella* spp in patients who are seriously ill without an alternative diagnosis, immunocompromised, nonresponsive to β-lactam antibiotics, have clinical features suggesting this diagnosis, or in outbreak setting. Urinary antigen testing is highly specific for serotype 1 but lacks specificity for other serotypes. Value and use vary by geographic region.
- Thoracentesis (if moderate to large effusion)

Aggravating Factors

- Age-related changes in pulmonary reserve
- Alcoholism
- Altered mental status
- Comorbid conditions that alter gag reflexes or ciliary transport
- COPD or other lung disease
- Heart disease
- Malnutrition
- Medications: Immunosuppressants, sedatives, anticholinergic or other agents that dry secretions, agents that decrease gastric pH
- Nasogastric tubes

Expected Organisms (in order of frequency of occurrence)

Community-Acquired:	*Nursing-Home–Acquired:*	*Hospital-Acquired:*
Streptococcus pneumoniae	*S pneumoniae*	Gram-negative bacteria
Respiratory viruses	Gram-negative bacteria	Anaerobes
Haemophilus influenzae	*Staphylococcus aureus*	Gram-positive bacteria
Gram-negative bacteria	Anaerobes	Fungi
Chlamydia pneumoniae	*H influenzae*	
Moraxella catarrhalis	Group B streptococcus	
Legionella spp	*Chlamydia pneumoniae*	
M tuberculosis		
Endemic fungi		

Supportive Management
- Chest percussion
- Inhaled β-adrenergic agonists
- Mechanical ventilation (if indicated)
- Oxygen as indicated
- Rehydration

Empiric Antibiotic Therapy (see **Table 46**)
Community-Acquired (oral route):
(2nd gen ceph or β-lact or FLQ*) ± macro if *Legionella* spp suspected
Community-Acquired with Hospitalization (oral or IV):
(2nd, 3rd, or 4th gen ceph or β-lact or FLQ*) ± erythromycin or other macro if *Legionella* spp suspected
Severe Community-Acquired with Hospitalization (IV):
Macro + ceftazidime or cefepime or other antipseudomonal agent
Nursing-Home Acquired (IV):
[(1st or 2nd gen ceph or antipseudomonal β-lact) + AG] ± pen G, clinda, or vanco
or 3rd or 4th gen ceph ± AG ± pen G, clinda, or vanco
or antipseudomonal β-lact + AG
or vanco + clinda + AG
For the oral route: see Community-Acquired (above) ± FLQ
Hospital-Acquired (IV):
[3rd or 4th gen ceph + clinda or pen G] ± AG
or antipseudomonal β-lact + AG or other antipseudomonal agent
or 1st or 2nd gen ceph + AG
or vanco + clinda + AG
or antipseudomonal β-lact + 2nd gen ceph
or β-lact + antipseudomonal agent
For hospital- or nursing-home-acquired pneumonia, a macro, tetracycline, or FLQ may be added or substituted when *Legionella* spp or *Mycobacterium pneumonia* is suspected.

*Refers to FLQ with enhanced activity against *S. pneumonia* (levofloxacin, sparfloxacin, moxifloxacin).
Note: AG = aminoglycoside; β-lact = β-lactam/ β-lactamase inhibitor; ceph = cephalosporin; clinda = clindamycin; FLQ = fluoroquinolone; gen = generation; macro = macrolide; pen G = penicillin G; vanco = vancomycin.

Note: The empiric use of vancomycin should be reserved for patients with a serious allergy to β-lactam antibiotics or for patients from environments in which methicillin-resistant *S aureus* is known to be a problem pathogen. For all cases, antimicrobial therapy should be individualized once Gram's stain or culture results are known.

URINARY TRACT INFECTION OR UROSEPSIS

Definition

Bacteriuria: Presence of significant number of bacteria without reference to symptoms

Symptomatic bacteriuria usually has signs of dysuria and increased frequency of urination; fever, chills, nausea may be present; pyuria ($>10^5$ cfu/mL) supports the diagnosis of UTI.

Asymptomatic bacteriuria is seen when the same organism(s) ($\geq 10^5$ cfu/mL) is found on 2 consecutive cultures in the absence of symptoms of a UTI; no treatment is necessary.

Risk Factors

- Abnormalities in function or anatomy of the urinary tract
- Catheterization or recent instrumentation
- Comorbid conditions (eg, diabetes mellitus, BPH)
- Female gender
- Limited functional status

Assessment and Evaluation

Choice is based on presenting symptoms and severity of illness.

- Urinalysis with culture (do not obtain specimen from catheter bag)
- Blood culture × 2
- BUN, creatinine, electrolytes
- CBC with differential

Expected Organisms

Noncatheterized Patients: Most common: *Escherichia coli, Proteus* spp, *Klebsiella* spp, *Providencia* spp, *Citrobacter* spp, *Enterobacter* spp, and *Pseudomonas aeruginosa* if recent antibiotic exposure, known colonization, or known institutional flora

Nursing-Home–Catheterized Patients: *Enterobacter* spp and gram-negative bacteria

Empiric Antibiotic Management

Duration should be at least 7–10 d.

Community-Acquired or Nursing-Home–Acquired Cystitis or Uncomplicated UTI (Oral Route): TMP/SMZ DS, cephalexin, ampicillin, or amoxicillin. Amoxicillin/clavulanic acid should be reserved for patients with sulfa allergy and in settings where β-lactam resistance is known. Fluoroquinolones should be reserved for patients with allergies to sulpha, β-lactams, or in settings where resistance is known.

Suspected Urosepsis (IV Route): Third-generation cephalosporin plus aminoglycoside, aztreonam, or fluoroquinolone ± aminoglycoside.

Vancomycin should be used in patients with severe β-lactam allergy.

UTI Prophylaxis

Generally not recommended because it leads to antibiotic resistance

HERPES ZOSTER ("SHINGLES")

Definition

Cutaneous vesicular eruptions followed by radicular pain secondary to the recrudescence of varicella zoster virus.

Clinical Manifestations

- An abrupt onset of pain along a specific dermatome (see **Figure 1**)
- Macular, erythematous rash after ~3 d which becomes vesicular and pustular (Tzanck cell test positive), crusts over and clears in 10–14 d
- Complications: post-herpetic neuralgia, visual loss or blindness if ophthalmic involvement

Pharmacologic Management

When started within 72 h of the rash's appearance, antiviral therapy decreases the severity and duration of the acute illness and possibly shortens the duration and reduces the risk of post-herpetic neuralgias. Corticosteroids may also decrease the risk and severity of post-herpetic neuralgia. (See p 115 for treatment of post-herpetic neuralgia.)

Table 41. Antiviral Treatments for Herpes Zoster			
Agent, Route	**Dosage**	**Formulations**	**Comment**
Acyclovir (*Zovirax*)			
Oral	800 mg 5 ×/d for 7–10 d	T: 400, 800; C: 200; S: 200 mg/5 mL	Reduce dose when CrCl* < 50 mL/min
IV**	7.5–10 mg/kg q 8 h for 7–10 d	500 mg/10 mL	
Famciclovir (*Famvir*)			
Oral	500 mg q 8 h for 7 d	T: 125, 250, 500	Reduce dose when CrCl* < 60 mL/min
Valacyclovir† (*Valtrex*)			
Oral	1000 mg q 8 h for 7 d	C: 500, 1000	Reduce dose when CrCl* < 50 mL/min

* The CrCl listed is the threshold below which the dose or frequency should be reduced. See alternative reference or the drug's package insert for detailed dosing guidelines.
** Use IV for serious illness, ophthalmic infection, or patients who cannot take oral medication.
† Preferred to po acyclovir; pro-drug of acyclovir with serum concentrations equal to IV.

INFLUENZA

Vaccine Prevention (ACIP Guidelines)

Yearly vaccination is recommended for all persons ≥ 65 years and all residents and staff of nursing homes, or residential or long-term-care facilities. Nursing-home residents admitted during the winter months after the completion of the vaccination program should be vaccinated at admission if they have not already been vaccinated. The influenza vaccine is contraindicated in persons with an anaphylactic hypersensitivity to eggs or any other component of the vaccine. Dose: 0.5 mL IM × 1 in the fall (Oct–Nov) for residents in the northern hemisphere.

Pharmacologic Prophylaxis and Treatment with Antiviral Agents
Indications:

- Prevention (during an influenza outbreak): persons who are not vaccinated, are immunodeficient, or may spread the virus
- Prophylaxis: during 2 wk required to develop antibodies for persons vaccinated after an outbreak of influenza A

- Reduction of symptoms, duration of illness when started within the first 48 h of symptoms
- During epidemic outbreaks in nursing homes

Duration: Treatment of symptoms: 3–5 d or for 24–48 h after symptoms resolve.
Prophylaxis during outbreak: Minimum 2 wk or until ~1 wk after end of outbreak.

Table 42. Antiviral Treatment of Influenza		
Agent	Formulation	Dosage
Amantadine (*Symmetrel*)	C: 100 mg; S: 50 mg/5 mL	100 mg po daily*
√ Oseltamivir (*Tamiflu*)**	C: 75 mg; S: 12 mg/mL	Treatment: 75 mg po bid × 5 d (75 mg po qd if CrCl 10–30 mL/min); not recommended if CrCl < 10 mL/min Prophylaxis: 75 mg po qd × ≥ 7 d up to 6 wk (75 mg po qod if CrCl 10–30 mL/min); not recommended if CrCl < 10 mL/min
√ Rimantadine (*Flumadine*)	T: 100 mg; S: 50 mg/5 mL	100 mg po qd for frail elderly and nursing-home residents 200 mg po qd for other adults, including those ≥ 65 yr Decrease dose to 100 mg if side effects appear
Zanamivir (*Relenza*)**†	Inh: 5 mg/blister	2 × 5–mg inhalations q 12 h × 5 d Give doses on 1st d at least 2 h apart

√ = preferred for treating older persons.
* Dose adjustments for renal function, CrCl (mL/min): ≥ 30 = 100 mg daily; 20–29 = 200 mg 2 ×/wk; 10–19 = 100 mg 3 ×/wk; < 10 = 200 mg alternating with 100 mg q 7 d.
** Must be started within 2 d of symptom onset.
† Do not use in patients with COPD or asthma.

INFECTIOUS TUBERCULOSIS

Tuberculosis (TB) in elderly patients may be the reactivation of old disease or a new infection due to exposure to an infected individual. Treatment recommendations differ; if a new infection is suspected or the patient has risk factors for resistant organisms, then bacterial sensitivities must be determined.

Risk or Reactivating Factors
- Chronic institutionalization
- Corticosteroid use
- Diabetes mellitus
- Malignancy
- Malnutrition
- Renal failure

Risk Factors for Resistant Organisms
- HIV infection
- Homelessness, institutionalization (other than a nursing home)
- IV drug abuse
- Origin from geographic regions with a high prevalence of resistance (New York, Mexico, Southeast Asia)
- Exposure to INH-resistant TB or history of failed chemotherapy
- Previous treatment for TB
- AFB-positive sputum smears after 2 mo of treatment
- Positive cultures after 4 mo of treatment

Diagnosis
- PPD with booster 5-TU subdermal; read in 48–72 h; repeat in 1–2 wk if negative (see **Table 43** for interpretation of test results)
- CXR

Treatment
Latent Infection:

Table 43. Identification of Patients at High Risk of Developing TB Who Would Benefit From Treatment of Latent Infection	
Population	**Minimum Induration Considered a Positive Test**
Low risk: testing generally not indicated	15 mm
Residents and employees of hospitals, nursing homes, and long-term facilities for elderly persons, residential facilities for AIDS patients, and homeless shelters Recent immigrants (< 5 yr) from high-prevalence countries Injection drug users Persons with silicosis, diabetes mellitus, chronic renal failure, leukemia, lymphoma, carcinoma of the head, neck, or lung, weight loss of ≥ 10%, gastrectomy or jejunoileal bypass	10 mm
Recent contact with TB patients Fibrotic changes on CXR consistent with prior TB Immunosuppressed (receiving the equivalent of ≥ 15 mg/d of prednisone for ≥ 1 mo) or organ transplants HIV-positive patients	5 mm

Table 44. Treatment of Latent Tuberculosis	
Drug	**Dosage and Duration**
INH*	5 mg/kg/d (maximum 300 mg/d) for 6 or 9 mo; or 15 mg/kg/d (maximum 900 mg/d) 2 × /wk with directly observed therapy (DOT) for 6 or 9 mo
RIF plus	10 mg/kg/d (maximum 600 mg/d)
PZA†	15–20 mg/kg/d (maximum 2 gm/d) daily for 2 mo
or RIF plus	10 mg/kg/d (maximum 600 mg/d) 2 × /wk with DOT for 2–3 mo
PZA†	50 mg/kg/d (maximum 4 gm/d) 2 × /wk with DOT for 2–3 mo
RIF	10 mg/kg/d (maximum 600 mg/d) for 4 mo

Note: INH = isoniazid; PZA = pyrazinamide; RIF = rifampin.

* The preferred treatment for patients not infected with HIV.

† Use the combination therapy with caution, as the 2-mo regimen has been associated with liver injury. Obtain a serum aminotransferase, and bilirubin at baseline and 2, 4, and 6 wk of treatment. For additional information, see *MMWR* 2001; 50(34):733–735 or http://ajrccm.atsjournals.org/cgi/content/full/161/4/S1/S221/DC1

Source: Data from: American Thoracic Society. Targeted tuberculin testing and treatment of latent tuberculosis. *Am J Respir Crit Care Med* 2000;161:S221–S247 (also available at www.atsjournal.org).

Active Infection:

Initial treatment options for adults with active *Mycobacterium tuberculosis* (note: INH = isoniazid; PZA = pyrazinamide; RIF = rifampin):

- Daily INH, RIF, and PZA × 8 wk, followed by 16 wk of INH and RIF daily or 2–3 times/wk. Add ethambutol or streptomycin to the initial regimen if area INH resistance rate is not documented to be < 4%; continue until susceptibility to INH and RIF are known.
- Daily INH, RIF, PZA, and ethambutol or streptomycin × 2 wk followed by all agents given 2 times/wk by daily observed therapy × 6 wk followed by INH and RIF 2 times/wk × 16 wk by daily observed therapy.
- INH, RIF, PZA, and ethambutol or streptomycin 3 times/wk for 6 mo by daily observed therapy.

Table 45. Dosing for Treatment Options for Active Tuberculosis				
Agent	Route	Daily	2/Wk	3/Wk
INH	po, IM	300 mg*	15 mg/kg*	15 mg/kg*
RIF	po, IM	600 mg**	600 mg**	600 mg**
PZA	po	1.5 g (< 50 kg) 2 g (51–74 kg) 2.5 g (≥ 75 kg)	2.0 g (< 50 kg) 2.5 g (51–74 kg) 3.0 g (≥ 75 kg)	2.0 g (< 50 kg) 2.5 g (51–74 kg) 3.0 g (≥ 75 kg)
Ethambutol	po	15–25 mg/kg†	50 mg/kg	30 mg/kg
Streptomycin	IM	10 mg/kg	—	—

* Maximums: daily = 300 mg; 2/wk = 900 mg; 3/wk = 900 mg.
** Maximums: daily = 600 mg; 2/wk = 600 mg; 3/wk= 600 mg.
† Maximum: daily = 2.5 g.

ANTIBIOTICS

Table 46. Antibiotics				
Class, *Subclass*, Antimicrobial	Route of Elimination (%)	Dosage	Adjust When CrCl* Is: (mL/min)	Formulations
β-Lactams				
Penicillins				
Amoxicillin (*Amoxil*)	K (80)	po: 250 mg–1 g q 8 h	< 50	T: film coated 500, 875 C: 250, 500 ChT: 125, 200, 250, 400 S: 125, 200, 250, 400 mg/5 mL
Ampicillin	K (90)	po: 250–500 mg q 6 h IM/IV: 1–2 g q 4–6 h	< 30	C: 250, 500 S: 125, 250 mg/5 mL Inj
Penicillin G	K L (30)	IV: 3–5 × 10⁶ U q 4–6 h IM: 0.6–2.4 × 10⁶ U q 6–12 h	< 30	Inj procaine for IM
Penicillin VK	K, L	po: 125–500 mg q 6 h		T: 250, 500

(continues)

Table 46. Antibiotics (cont.)				
Class, *Subclass*, Antimicrobial	Route of Elimination (%)	Dosage	Adjust When CrCl* Is: (mL/min)	Formulations
Antipseudomonal Penicillins				
Carbenicillin indanyl sodium (*Geocillin*)	K (80–99)	po: 382–764 mg q 6 h	< 50	S: 125, 250 mg/5 mL T: 382
Piperacillin (*Pipracil*)	K, F	IM: 1–2 g q 8–12 h IV: 2–4 g q 6–8 h	< 40	Inj
Ticarcillin (*Ticar*)	K	IM, IV: 1–4 g q 4–6 h	< 60	Inj
Antistaphylococcal Penicillins				
Dicloxacillin (*Dycill, Pathocil*)	K (56–70)	PO: 125–500 mg q 6 h	NA	C: 125, 250, 500; S: 62.5 mg/5 mL
Nafcillin	L	IM: 500 mg q 4–6 h IV: 500 mg–2 g q 4–6 h	NA	Inj
Oxacillin (*Bactocill*)	K	po: 500 mg–1 g q 4–6 h IM, IV: 250 mg–2 g q 6–12 h	< 10	C: 250, 500 S: 250 mg/5 mL Inj
Monobactam (antipseudomonal)				
Aztreonam (*Azactam*)	K (70)	IM: 500 mg–1 g q 8–12 h IV: 500 mg–2 g q 6–12 h	< 30	Inj
Carbapenem (antipseudomonal)				
Imipenem-Cilastatin (*Primaxin*)	K (70)	IM: 500 mg–1 g q 8–12 h IV: 500 mg–2 g q 6–12 h	< 70	Inj
Meropenem (*Merrem IV*)	K (75), L (25)	IV: 1 g q 8 h	≤ 50	Inj
Penicillinase-resistant Penicillins				
Amoxicillin– Clavulanate (*Augmentin*)	K	po: 250 mg q 8 h, 500 mg q 12 h, 875 mg q 12 h	< 30	T: 250, 500, 875 ChT: 125, 200, 250, 400 S: 125, 200, 250, 400 mg/5 mL
Ampicillin–Sulbactam (*Unasyn*)	K (85)	IM, IV: 1–2 g q 6–8 h	< 30	Inj
Penicillinase-resistant and Antipseudomonal Penicillins				
Piperacillin– Tazobactam (*Zosyn*)	K	IV: 3.375 g q 6 h	< 40	Inj
Ticarcillin– Clavulanate (*Timentin*)	K, L	IV: 3 g q 4–6 h	< 60	Inj
First-Generation Cephalosporins				
Cefadroxil (*Duricef*)	K (90)	po: 500 mg–1 g q 12 h	< 50	C: 500; T: 1 g S: 125, 250, 500 mg/ 5 mL
Cefazolin (*Ancef, Kefzol*)	K (80–100)	IM, IV: 500 mg–2 g q 8 h	< 55	Inj
Cephalexin (*Keflex*)	K (80–100)	po: 250 mg–1 g q 6 h	< 40	C: 250, 500 T: 250, 500; 1 g S: 125, 250 mg/5 mL
Cephalothin (*Keflin*)	K (50–75)	IM, IV: 500 mg–2 g q 4–6 h	< 50	Inj
Cephapirin (*Cefadyl*)	K (60–85)	IM, IV: 1–3 g q 6 h	< 10	Inj

Table 46. Antibiotics (cont.)				
Class, *Subclass*, Antimicrobial	Route of Elimination (%)	Dosage	Adjust When CrCl* Is: (mL/min)	Formulations
Cephradine (*Anspor*)	K (80–90)	po, IM, IV: 500 mg–2 g q 6 h	< 20	C: 250, 500 T: 1 g S: 125, 250 mg/5 mL Inj
Second-Generation Cephalosporins				
Cefaclor (*Ceclor*)	K (80)	po: 250–500 mg q 8 h	< 50	C: 250, 500 S: 125, 187, 250, 375 mg/5 mL T: ER 375, 500
Cefamandole (*Mandol*)	K	IM, IV: 1–3 g q 6 h	< 80	Inj
Cefmetazole (*Zefazone*)	K (85)	IV: 2 g q 6–12 h	< 90	Inj
Cefotetan (*Cefotan*)	K (80)	IM, IV: 1–3 g q 12 h or 1–2 g q 24 h (UTI)	< 30	Inj
Cefoxitin (*Mefoxin*)	K (85)	IM, IV: 1–2 g q 6–8 h	< 50	Inj
Cefprozil (*Cefzil*)	K (60–70)	po: 250–500 mg q 12–24 h	< 30	T: 250, 500 S: 125, 250 mg/5 mL
Cefuroxime axetil (*Ceftin*)	K (66–100)	po: 125–500 mg q 12 h IM, IV: 750 mg–1.5 g q 6 h	< 20	T: 125, 250, 500 S: 125, 150 mg/5 mL Inj
Loracarbef (*Lorabid*)	K	po: 200–400 mg q 12–24 h	< 50	C: 200, 400 S: 100, 200 mg/5 mL
Third-Generation Cephalosporins				
Cefdinir (*Omnicef*)	K	po: 300 mg bid or 600 qd × 10 d	< 30	C: 300 S: 125 mg/5 mL
Cefixime (*Suprax*)	K (50)	po: 400 mg q 24 h	< 60	T: 200, 400 S: 100 mg/5 mL
Cefoperazone (*Cefobid*)	L, K (25)	IM, IV: 1–2 g q 12 h	Adjust in cirrhosis	Inj
Cefotaxime (*Claforan*)	K, L	IM, IV: 1–2 g q 6–12 h	< 20	Inj
Cefpodoxime (*Vantin*)	K (80)	po: 100–400 mg q 12 h	< 30	T: 100, 250 S: 50, 100 mg/5 mL
Ceftazidime (*Ceptaz, Fortaz*)	K	IM, IV: 500 mg–2 g q 8–12 h UTI: 250–500 mg q 12 h	< 50	Inj
Ceftibuten (*Cedax*)	K (65–70)	po: 400 mg q 24 h	< 50	C: 400 S: 100, 200 mg/5 mL
Ceftizoxime (*Cefizox*)	K (100)	IM, IV: 500 mg–2 g q 4–12 h	< 80	Inj
Ceftriaxone (*Rocephin*)	K (33–65)	IM, IV: 1–2 g q 12–24 h	NA	Inj
Fourth-Generation Cephalosporins				
Cefepime (*Maxipime*)	K (85)	IV: 500 mg–2 g q 12 h	< 60	Inj
Aminoglycosides				
Amikacin (*Amikin*)	K (95)	IM, IV: 15–20 mg/kg/d divided q 12–24 h; 15–20 mg/kg q 24–48 h		Inj

(*continues*)

Table 46. Antibiotics (cont.)				
Class, *Subclass*, Antimicrobial	Route of Elimination (%)	Dosage	Adjust When CrCl* Is: (mL/min)	Formulations
Gentamicin (*Garamycin*)	K (95)	IM, IV: 2–5 mg/kg/d divided q 12–24 h; 5–7 mg/kg q 24–48 h		Inj ophth sus, oint
Streptomycin	K (90)	IM, IV: 10 mg/kg/d not to exceed 750 mg/d	< 50	Inj
Tobramycin (*Nebcin*)	K (95)	IM, IV: 2–5 mg/kg/d divided q 12–24 h; 5–7 mg/kg q 24–48 h		Inj ophth sus, oint
Macrolides				
Azithromycin (*Zithromax*)	L	po: 500 mg day 1, then 250 mg IV: 500 mg qd	NA	C: 250 S: 100, 200 mg/5 mL, 1 g (single-dose pk) T: 600
Clarithromycin (*Biaxin, Biaxin XL*)	L, K (20–30)	po: 250–500 mg q 12 h ER: 1000 mg q 24 h	< 30	S: 125, 250 mg/5 mL T: 250, 500 ER: 500
Dirithromycin (*Dynabac*)	L, F	po: 500 mg qd with food	NA	T: 250
Erythromycin	L	po: Base: 333 mg q 8 h Estolate, stearate or base: 250–500 mg q 6–12 h Ethylsuccinate: 400–800 mg q 6–12 h IV: 15–20 mg/kg/d divided q 6 h	NA	Base: C, T: 250, 333, 500 Estolate: 250 S: 125, 250 mg/5 mL T: 500 Ethylsuccinate: S: 100, 200, 400 mg/5 mL T: 400 ChT: 200 Stearate: T: 250, 500 Inj
Quinolones				
Cinoxacin (*Cinobac*)	K (60)	po: 500 mg bid	< 80	C: 250, 500
Ciprofloxacin (*Cipro*)	K (30–50), L, F (20–40)	po: 250–750 mg q 12 h IV: 200–400 mg q 12 h ophth: see **Table 81 note**	po: < 50 IV: < 30	T: 100, 250, 500, 750 S: 250 mg/5 mL, 500 mg/5 mL ophth sol: 3.5 mg/5 mL Inj
Enoxacin (*Penetrex*)	K, L (15–20)	po: 200 mg q 12 h × 7 d or 400 mg q 12 h × 14 d	≤ 30	T: 200, 400
Gatifloxacin (*Tequin*)	K (95), F (5)	po, IV: 200–400 mg qd × 7–10 d	< 40	T: 200, 400 Inj
Gemifloxacin (*Factive*)	K, L, F	po: 320 mg qd	≤40	T: 320 mg
Levofloxacin (*Levaquin*)	K	po, IV: 250–500 mg q 24 h	< 50	T: 250, 500
Lomefloxacin (*Maxaquin*)	K	po: 400 mg q 24 h	< 40	T: 400
Moxifloxacin (*Avelox*)	L (~55), F (25), K (20)	po: 400 mg q 24 h	NA	T: 400
Norfloxacin (*Noraxin*)	K (30), F (30)	po: 400 mg q 12 h ophth: see **Table 81 note**	< 30	T: 400 ophth: 0.3%

Table 46. Antibiotics (cont.)				
Class, *Subclass*, Antimicrobial	Route of Elimination (%)	Dosage	Adjust When CrCl* Is: (mL/min)	Formulations
Ofloxacin (*Roxin*)	K	po, IV: 200–400 mg q 12–24 h ophth: see **Table 81 note**	< 50	T: 200, 300, 400 ophth: 0.3% Inj
Sparfloxacin (*Zagam*)	L	po: 400 mg day 1, then 200 mg q 24 h	< 50	T: 200
Trovafloxacin (*Trovan*)	L	po, IV: 200 mg q 24 h × 10–14 d	NA	T: 100, 200 Inj
Tetracyclines				
Doxycycline (eg, *Vibramycin*)	K (25), F (30)	po, IV: 100–200 mg/d given q 12–24 h	NA	C: 50, 100 T: 50, 100 S:25 mg/5 mL, 50 mg/5 mL Inj
Minocycline (*Minocin*)	K	po, IV: 200 mg × 1, 100 mg q 12 h	NA	C: 50, 100 . S: 50 mg/5 mL Inj
Tetracycline	K (60)	po, IV: 250–500 mg q 6–12 h	NA	C: 100, 250, 500 T: 250, 500 S: 125 mg/5 mL ophth: oint, sus topical: oint, sol
Other Antibiotics				
Chloramphenicol (*Chloromycetin*)	L (90)	po, IV: 50 mg/kg/d given q 6 h; maximum: 4 g/d		C: 250 topical ophth Inj
Clindamycin (*Cleocin*)	L (90)	po: 150–450 mg q 6–8 h; maximum: 1.8 g/d IM, IV: 1.2–1.8 g/d given q 8–12 h; maximum: 3.6 g/d	NA	C: 75, 150, 300 S: 75 mg/5 mL crm, vaginal: 2% gel, topical: 1% Inj
Co-trimoxazole (TMP/SMZ, *Bactrim*)	K, L	Doses based on the trimethoprim component: po: 1 double-strength tablet q 12 h; sepsis: 20 TMP/kg/d given q 6 h	≤ 50	T: SMZ 400; TMP 80 double-strength: SMZ 800; TMP 160 S: SMZ 200; TMP 40 mg/5 mL Inj
Linezolid (*Zyvox*)	L (65), K (30)	po: 400–600 mg q 12 h IV: 600 mg q 12 h	NA	T: 400, 600 S: 100 mg/5 mL Inj
Metronidazole (*Flagyl*, *MetraGel*)	L (30–60), K (20–40), F (6–15)	po: 250–750 mg q 6–8 h Vaginal: 1 applicator full (375 mg) qhs or bid Topical: Apply bid	≤ 10	T: 250, 500 ER: 750 C: 375 gel, topical: 0.75% (30 g) gel, vaginal: 0.75% (70 g) Inj
Nitrofurantoin (*Macrodantin*)	L (60), K (40)	po: 50–100 mg q 6 h	Do not use if < 40	C: 25, 50, 100 S: 25 mg/5 mL

(*continues*)

Class, *Subclass*, Antimicrobial	Route of Elimination (%)	Dosage	Adjust When CrCl* Is: (mL/min)	Formulations
Quinupristin/ dalfopristin (*Synercid*)	L, B, F (75), K (15–19)	Vancomycin-resistant *E faecium*: IV: 7.5 mg/ kg q 8 h Complicated skin or skin structure infection: 7.5 mg/kg q 12 h	NA	Inj
Vancomycin (*Vancocin*)	K (80–90)	po: *C difficile*: 125–500 mg q 6–8 h IV: 500 mg–1 g q 8–24 h Peak: 20–40 µg/mL Trough: 5–10 µg/mL		C: 125, 250 Inj
Antifungals				
Amphotericin B (*Fungizone*)	K	IV: test dose: 1 mg infused over 20–30 min; if tolerated, initial therapeutic dose is 0.25 mg/kg; the daily dose can be increased by 0.25-mg/kg increments on each subsequent day until the desired daily dose is reached Maintenance dose: IV: 0.25–1 mg/kg/d or 1.5 mg/kg qod; do not exceed 1.5 mg/kg/d	**	topical: crm, lot, oint 3% Inj
Amphotericin B Lipid Complex (*Abelcet*)	K	2.5–5 mg/k/d as a single infusion		Inj
Amphotericin B Liposomal (*AmBisome*)	K	3–5 mg/k/d infused over 1–2 h		Inj
Amphotericin B Colloidal Dispersion (*Amphotec*)	K	3–4 mg/k/d infused at 1 mg/k/h; maximum dosage 7.5 mg/kg/d		Inj
Caspofungin (*Cancidas*)	L	Initial: 70 mg infused over 1 h, then 50 mg/d over 1 h	—	Inj
Fluconazole (*Diflucan*)	K (80)	po, IV: first dose 50– 400 mg, then 50– 400 mg qd for 14 d–12 wk, depending on indication. Vaginal candidiasis: 150 mg as a single dose	< 50	T: 50, 100, 150, 200 S: 10 and 40 mg/mL Inj
Flucytosine (*Ancobon*)	K (75–90)	po: 50–150 mg/kg/d divided q 6 h	< 40	C: 250, 500

Table 46. Antibiotics (cont.)

Table 46. Antibiotics (cont.)				
Class, *Subclass*, Antimicrobial	Route of Elimination (%)	Dosage	Adjust When CrCl* Is: (mL/min)	Formulations
Griseofulvin (*Fulvicin P/G, Grifulvin V*)	L	po: Microsize: 500–1000 mg/d in single or divided doses Ultramicrosize: 330–375 mg/d in single or divided doses Duration based on indication	NA	Microsize: S: 125 mg/5 mL T: 250, 500 Ultramicrosize: T: 125, 165, 250, 330
Itraconazole (*Sporanox*)	L	po: 200–400 mg/d; doses > 200 mg/d should be divided. Life-threatening infections: loading dose: 200 mg tid (600 mg/d) should be given for the first 3 d of therapy IV: 200 mg bid × 4 d, then 200 mg qd	< 30	C: 100 S: 100 mg/10 mL Inj
Ketoconazole (*Nizoral*)	L, F	po: 200–400 mg qd shp: 2/wk × 4 wk with at least 3 d between each shp Topical: apply qd–bid	NA	crm: 2% shp: 2% T: 200
Miconazole (*Monistat IV*)	L, F	IT: 20 mg q 1–2 d IV: initial: 200 mg, then 1.2–3.6 g/d divided q 8 h for up to 2 wk	NA	Inj
Terbinafine (*Lamisil*)	L, K	po: 250 mg/d × 6–12 wk for superficial mycoses; 250–500 mg/d for up to 16 mo Topical: apply 1–2 times/d for a maximum of 4 wk	< 50	T: 250 mg crm: 1% topical S: 1%
Voriconazole (*VFEND*)	L	IV: loading dose 6 mg/kg q 12 h for 2 doses, then 4 mg/k q 12 h po: > 40 kg: 200 mg q 12 h; ≤ 40 kg: 100 mg q 12 h If on phenytoin, IV: 5 mg/kg q 12 h, and po: > 40 kg: 400 mg q 12 h; ≤ 40 kg: 200 mg q 12 h	< 50 (IV only)	Inj T: 50, 200 mg

Note: NA = not applicable.
* The CrCl listed is the threshold below which the dose or frequency should be adjusted. See alternative reference or the drug package insert for detailed dosing guidelines.
** Adjust dose if decreased renal function is due to the drug, or give every other day.

MALNUTRITION

DEFINITION
There is no uniformly accepted definition of malnutrition in older persons. Some commonly used definitions include the following:

Community-Dwelling Men and Women
- Involuntary weight loss (eg, $\geq$ 10 lb over 6 months, $\geq$ 4% over 1 yr)
- Abnormal body mass index (eg, BMI > 27; BMI < 22)
- Hypoalbuminemia (eg, $\leq$ 3.8 g/dL)
- Hypocholesterolemia (eg, < 160 mg/dL)
- Specific vitamin or micronutrient deficiencies (eg, vitamin B_{12})

Hospitalized Patients
- Dietary intake (eg, < 50% of estimated needed caloric intake)
- Hypoalbuminemia (eg, < 3.5 g/dL)
- Hypocholesterolemia (eg, < 160 mg/dL)

Nursing-Home Patients (Triggered by the Minimum Data Set)
- Weight loss of $\geq$ 5% in past 30 d; $\geq$ 10% in 180 d
- Dietary intake of < 75% at most meals

EVALUATION
Multidimensional Assessment
In the absence of valid nutrition screening instruments, clinicians should focus on whether the following issues may be affecting nutritional status:
- Economic barriers to securing food
- Availability of sufficiently high-quality food
- Dental problems that prohibit ingesting high-quality food
- Medical illnesses that
  - interfere with digestion or absorption of food
  - increase nutritional requirements
  - require dietary restrictions (eg, low-sodium diet or npo)
- Functional disability that interferes with shopping, preparing meals, or feeding
- Food preferences or cultural beliefs that interfere with adequate food intake
- Poor appetite
- Depressive symptoms

Anthropometrics
Weight on each visit and yearly height (see p 1)

Biochemical Markers
Serum Proteins: All may drop precipitously because of trauma, sepsis, or major infection.
- Albumin (half-life 18–20 d) has prognostic value in all settings.
- Transferrin (half-life 7 d)
- Prealbumin (half-life 48 h) may be valuable in monitoring nutritional recovery.

Serum Cholesterol (Low or Falling Levels): Has prognostic value in all settings but may not be nutritionally mediated.

MANAGEMENT
Calculating Basic Energy (Caloric) and Fluid Requirements
- WHO energy estimates for adults aged 60 yr and older:
  - Women (10.5) (weight in kg) + 596
  - Men (13.5) (weight in kg) + 487
- Harris-Benedict energy requirement equations:
  - Women 655 + (9.6) (weight in kg) + (1.7) (height in cm) − (4.7) (age in yr)
  - Men 66 + (13.7) (weight in kg) + (5.0) (height in cm) − (6.8) (age in yr)

Depending on activity and physiologic stress levels, these basic requirements may need to be increased (eg, 25% for sedentary or mild, 50% for moderate, and 100% for intense or severe activity or stress).

- Fluid requirements for older persons without cardiac or renal disease are approximately 30 mL/kg of body weight/d.

Appetite Stimulants
- No drugs are FDA approved for weight loss in older persons.
- Dronabinol and megestrol acetate have been effective in promoting weight gain in younger adults with specific conditions (eg, AIDS, cancer).
- A minority of patients receiving mirtazapine report appetite stimulation and weight gain.
- All drugs used for appetite have substantial potential side effects.

Oral and Enteral Formulas
Many formulas are available (see **Table 47**). Read the content labels and choose on the basis of calories/mL, protein, fiber, lactose, and fluid load.
- Oral: Many (eg, *Carnation Instant Breakfast, Health Shake*) are milk-based and provide approximately 1.0–1.5 calories/mL.
- Enteral: Commercial preparations have between 0.5 and 2.0 calories/mL; most contain no milk (lactose) products. For patients who need fluid restriction, the higher concentrated formulas may be valuable, but they may cause diarrhea. Because of reduced kidney function with aging, some recommend that protein should contribute no more than 20% of the formula's total calories. If formula is sole source of nutrition, consider one that contains fiber (25 g/d is optimal).

Table 47. Examples of Lactose-Free Oral and Enteral Products							
Product	Kcal/mL	mOsm	Protein (g/L)	Water (mL/L)	Na (mEq/L)	K (mEq/L)	Fiber (g/L)
Oral—low residue							
Boost Basic	1.06	650	37.0	850	37.0	41.0	0
Boost Plus	1.50	670	61.0	780	37.0	38.0	< 1
Ensure	1.06	470	37.3	845	37.0	40.0	0
Ensure Plus	1.50	690	54.9	769	46.0	40.0	0
Nu Basics	1.00	480	35.0	842	38.0	32.0	0
Nu Basics Plus	1.50	620	42.4	776	50.8	48.0	0

(*continues*)

Table 47. Examples of Lactose-Free Oral and Enteral Products (cont.)							
Product	Kcal/mL	mOsm	Protein (g/L)	Water (mL/L)	Na (mEq/L)	K (mEq/L)	Fiber (g/L)
Oral—high fiber (can also be given enterally)							
Boost with Fiber	1.00	480	43.0	850	31.0	41.0	12.0
Ensure Fiber with FOS	1.06	500	36.0	780	37.0	40.0	12.0
Oral—clear liquid							
Citrisource	0.76	700	37.0	876	10.0	1.6	0
Resource	1.06	430	33.0	842	24.0	1.3	0
Oral—diabetes formulations							
Choicedm beverage	0.93	400	39.0	850	37.0	46.5	11
Glucerna shake	0.93	530	40.0	800	37.0	43.0	12
Enlive	1.25	671	40.0	764	11.6	4.1	0
Enteral—diabetes formulations							
Choicedm TF	1.06	300	45.0	850	37.0	47.0	14.4
Glucerna	1.00	355	41.8	853	40.5	40.2	14.4
Enteral—low residue							
Isocal	1.06	270	34.0	850	23.0	34.0	0
Osmolite	1.06	300	37.2	841	28.0	26.0	0
Nutren 1.0	1.00	315	40.0	852	38.1	32.0	0
Enteral—low volume							
Deliver	2.00	640	75.0	710	35.0	43.0	0
Nutren 2.0	2.00	745	80.0	700	56.5	49.2	0
TwoCal HN	2.00	730	83.5	701	63.5	62.7	0
Enteral—high fiber							
Jevity	1.06	310	44.4	830	40.0	40.0	14.4
Ultracal	1.06	310	44.0	850	40.0	41.0	14.4
Nutren 1.0 with fiber	1.00	320	40.0	840	38.1	32.0	14.0

Important Drug-Enteral Interactions

- Soybean formulas increase fecal elimination of thyroxine; time administration of thyroxine and enteral nutrition as far apart as possible.
- Enteral feedings reduce absorption of phenytoin; administer phenytoin at least 2 h following a feeding and delay feeding at least 2 h after phenytoin is administered; monitor levels and adjust doses, as necessary.
- Check with pharmacy about suitability and best way to administer sustained-release, enteric-coated, and micro-encapsulated products (eg, omeprazole, lansoprazole, diltiazem, fluoxetine, verapamil).

Tips for Successful Tube Feeding

- Gastrostomy tube feeding may be either intermittent or continuous.
- Jejunostomy tube feedings must be continuous.
- Continuous tube feeding is associated with less frequent diarrhea but with higher rates of tube clogging.
- To prevent clogging and to provide additional free water, flushing with at least 30–60 cc of water 4–6 times a day is recommended. Sometimes sugar-free carbonated beverages, cranberry juice, or meat tenderizer can restore patency to clogged tubes.
- Diarrhea, which occurs in 5%–30% of persons receiving enteral feeding, may be related to the osmolality of the formula, the rate of delivery, high sorbitol content in

liquid medications (eg, APAP, lithium, oxybutynin, furosemide), or other patient-related factors such as antibiotic use or impaired absorption.
- To help prevent aspiration, maintain a 30-degree elevation of the head of the bed during continuous feeding and for at least 2 h following bolus feedings.
- Do not administer bulk-forming laxatives (eg, methylcellulose or psyllium) through feeding tubes.
- Check gastric residual volume before each bolus feeding and hold feeding for at least 1 h if residual is more than half of previous feeding volume. Metoclopramide (*Reglan*) 5–10 mg [5 mg/5 mL] qid may be useful for high gastric residual volume problems once mechanical obstruction has been excluded.

Parenteral Nutrition
Indicated in those with digestive dysfunction precluding enteral feeding. Delivers protein as amino acids, carbohydrate as dextrose, and fat as lipid emulsions.
Peripheral Parenteral Nutrition: For short-term use. Requires rotation of peripheral IV site every 72 h. Solution osmolarity of less than 900 mOsm/L is recommended to reduce risk of phlebitis (see **Table 48**).
Total Parenteral Nutrition: Must be administered through a central catheter, which may be inserted peripherally.

Table 48. Caloric Value and Osmolarity of Parenteral Solutions		
Solution	Caloric Value (Kcal/L)	Osmolarity (mOsm/L)
Dextrose (%)		
5	170	250
10	340	500
20	680	1000
Lipid emulsions (%)		
10	1100	230
20	2200	330–340

Source: Bçikston SJ. In: Ewald GA, McKenzie CR. *Manual of Medical Therapeutics*. 28th ed. Boston: Little, Brown;1995:36. Copyright © 1995 by Little, Brown & Company. Reprinted with permission.

SHOULDER PAIN: DIFFERENTIAL DIAGNOSIS AND TREATMENT

Rotator Cuff Tendinitis, Subacromial Bursitis, or Rotator Tendon Impingement on Clavicle

Dull ache radiating to upper arm. Painful arc (on abduction 60–120 degrees and external rotation) is characteristic. Also can be distinguished by applying resistance against active range of motion while immobilizing the neck with hand.

Treatment: Identify and eliminate provocative, repetitive injury (eg, avoid overhead reaching). A brief period of rest and immobilization with a sling may be helpful. Pain control with APAP or NSAIDs (**Table 49**), home exercises or PT (especially assisted range of motion and wall walking), and corticosteroid injections may be useful.

Rotator Cuff Tears

Mild to complete; characterized by diminished shoulder movement. If severe, patients do not have full range of active or passive motion. The "drop arm" sign (the inability to maintain the arm in an abducted 90-degree position) indicates supraspinatus and infraspinatus tear. Weakness of external rotation (elbows flexed, thumbs up with examiner's hands outside patient's elbows; patient is asked to resist inward pressure) is common. MRI establishes diagnosis.

Treatment: If due to injury, a brief period of rest and immobilization with a sling may be helpful. Pain control with APAP or NSAIDs (**Table 49**), home exercises or PT (especially assisted range of motion and wall walking) may be useful. If no improvement after 6–8 wk of conservative measures, consider surgical repair.

Bicipital Tendinitis

Pain felt on anterior lateral aspect of shoulder, tenderness in the groove between greater and lesser tuberosities of the humerus. Pain is produced on resisted flexion of shoulder, flexion of the elbow, or supination (external rotation) of the hand and wrist with the elbow flexed at the side.

Treatment: Identify and eliminate provocative, repetitive activities (eg, avoid overhead reaching). A period of rest (at least 7 d with no lifting) and corticosteroid injections are major components of therapy. After rest period, PT should focus on stretching biceps tendon (eg, putting arm on doorframe and hyperextending shoulder, with some external rotation).

Frozen Shoulder (Adhesive Capsulitis)

Loss of passive external (lateral) rotation, abduction, and internal rotation of the shoulder to less than 90 degrees. Usually follows three phases: painful (freezing) phase lasting wks to a few mo; adhesive (stiffening) phase lasting 4–12 mo; resolution phase lasting 6–24 mo.

Treatment: Avoid rest and begin PT and home exercises for stretching the arm in flexion, horizontal adduction, and internal and external rotation. Corticosteroid injections may reduce pain and permit more aggressive PT. Consider surgical manipulation under anesthesia or arthroscopic dilation of capsule.

BACK PAIN: DIFFERENTIAL DIAGNOSIS AND TREATMENT

Acute Lumbar Strain (Low Back Pain Syndrome)

Acute pain frequently precipitated by heavy lifting or exercise. Pain may be central or more prominent on one side and may radiate to sacroiliac region and buttocks. Pain is aggravated by motion, standing, and prolonged sitting, and relieved by rest. Sciatic pain may be present even when neurologic examination is normal.

Treatment: Most can continue normal activities. If a patient obtains symptomatic relief from bed rest, generally 1–2 d lying in a semi-Fowler position or on side with the hips and knees flexed with pillow between legs will suffice. Treat muscle spasm with the application of ice, preferably in a massage over the muscles in spasm. APAP or NSAIDs **(Table 49)** can be used to control pain. As pain diminishes, encourage patient to begin isometric abdominal and lower-extremity exercises. Symptoms often recur. Education on back posture, lifting precautions, and abdominal muscle strengthening may help prevent recurrences.

Acute Disk Herniation

Over 90% of cases occur at L4–L5 or L5–S1 levels, resulting in unilateral impairment of ankle reflex, toe and ankle dorsiflexion, and pain (commonly sciatic) on straight leg raising (can be tested from sitting position by leg extension). Pain is acute in onset and varies considerably with changes in position.

Treatment: Initially same as acute lumbar strain (above). If unresponsive, administer epidural injection of a combination of a long-acting corticosteroid with an epidural anesthetic. Consider surgery if recurrence or persistence with neurologic signs beyond 6–8 wk after conservative treatment. The value of epidural injections and surgery for pain without neurologic signs is controversial. (See **Table 2** and **Table 3**.)

Osteoarthritis and Chronic Disk Degeneration

Characterized by aching pain aggravated by motion and relieved by rest. Occasionally, hypertrophic spurring in a facet joint may cause unilateral radiculopathy with sciatica. *Treatment:* Identify and eliminate provocative activities. Education on back posture, lifting precautions, and abdominal muscle strengthening. APAP or NSAIDs **(Table 49)**. Corticosteroid injections may be useful. Consider opioids and other pain treatment modalities for chronic refractory pain (see p 121).

Unstable Lumbar Spine

Severe, sudden, short-lasting, frequently recurrent pain often brought on by sudden, unguarded movements. Pain is reproduced upon moving from the flexed to the erect position. Pain is usually relieved by lying supine or on side. Impingement on nerve roots by spurs from facet joints or herniated disks can cause similar complaints, although symptoms in these conditions usually worsen as time passes. Symptoms can mimic disk herniation or degeneration, or osteoarthritis. Lumbar flexion x-rays can be diagnostic. *Treatment:* Surgery only in severe cases.

Lumbar Spinal Stenosis

Symptoms increase on spinal extension (eg, with prolonged standing, walking downhill, lying prone) and decrease with spinal flexion (eg, sitting, bending forward while walking, lying in the flexed position). Only symptom may be fatigue or pain in legs when walking (pseudo-claudication). May have immobility of lumbar spine, pain with straight leg raises, weakness of muscles innervated by L4 through S1 (see **Table 2**). Over 4 yr, 15% improve, 15% deteriorate, and 70% remain stable.

Treatment: APAP or NSAIDs (**Table 49**) and exercises to reduce lumbar lordosis are sometimes beneficial. Corticosteroid injections may be useful. Surgical intervention is more effective than conservative treatment in relieving moderate or severe symptoms; however, recurrence of pain several years after surgery is common.

Vertebral Compression Fracture

Immediate onset of severe pain; worse with sitting or standing; sometimes relieved by lying down.

Treatment: See Osteoporosis (p 116). Bed rest, analgesia, and mobilization as tolerated. Calcitonin may provide symptomatic improvement. May require hospitalization to control symptoms. Percutaneous vertebroplasty or kyphoplasty may be effective for pain relief in refractory cases (see p 116).

Nonrheumatic Pain (eg, Tumors, Aneurysms)

Gradual onset, steadily expanding, often unrelated to position and not relieved by lying down. Night pain when lying down is characteristic. Upper motor neuron signs may be present. Involvement is usually in thoracic and upper lumbar spine.

HIP PAIN: DIFFERENTIAL DIAGNOSIS AND TREATMENT

Trochanteric Bursitis

Pain in lateral aspect of the hip that usually worsens when patient sits on a hard chair, lies on the affected side, or rises from a chair or bed; pain may improve with walking. Local tenderness over greater trochanter is often present, and pain is often reproduced on resisted abduction of the leg or internal rotation of the hip. However, trochanteric bursitis does not produce limited range of motion, pain on range of motion, pain in the groin, or radicular signs.

Treatment: Identify and eliminate provocative activities. Check for leg length discrepancy, prescribe orthotics if appropriate. Injection of a combination of a long-acting corticosteroid with an anesthetic is most effective treatment.

Osteoarthritis

"Boring" quality pain in the hip, often in the groin, and sometimes referred to the back or knee with stiffness after rest. Passive motion is restricted in all directions if disease is fairly advanced. In early disease, pain in the groin on internal rotation of the hip is characteristic.

Treatment: See Osteoarthritis (p 99). Elective total hip replacement is indicated for patients who have radiographic evidence of joint damage and moderate to severe persistent pain or disability, or both, that is not substantially relieved by an extended course of nonsurgical management.

National Institutes of Health Consensus Development Conference Statement September 12–14, 1994 (reviewed 1998).

Hip Fracture

Sudden onset, usually after a fall, with inability to walk or bear weight, frequently radiating to groin or knee.

Treatment: Treatment is surgical with open reduction and internal fixation, hemiarthroplasty, or total hip replacement, depending on site of fracture and amount of displacement. For patients who were nonambulatory prior to the fracture, conservative management is an option.

Nonrheumatic Pain
Referred pain from viscera, radicular pain from the lower spine, avascular necrosis, Paget's disease, metastasis.

CARPAL TUNNEL SYNDROME
Definition
Painful tingling or hypoesthesia, or both, in one or both hands in distribution innervated by median nerve

Causes
- repetitive activities
- diabetes
- thyroid disease
- amyloidosis
- rheumatoid arthritis
- space-occupying lesions (eg, lymphoma)
- trauma (eg, Colles' fracture)

Evaluation and Assessment
Physical Examination:
- Decreased sensation in palm, thumb, index finger, middle finger, and thumb side of ring finger
- Weak handgrip
- Tapping over the median nerve at the wrist causes pain to shoot from wrist to hand (Tinel's sign)
- Acute flexion of wrist for 60 sec (Phalen's test) should also result in pain

Laboratory Studies:
- Fasting glucose
- TSH
- Nerve conduction velocity testing confirms diagnosis

Treatment
Nonpharmacologic:
- Redesign work or leisure processes to avoid repetitive movements
- Splinting in neutral position, especially at night
- Surgery (more effective than splinting)

Pharmacologic:
- Injectable corticosteroids, eg, methylprednisolone 15 mg (more effective than oral)
- Oral corticosteroids, eg, prednisone 20 mg/d for 1 wk followed by 10 mg/d for a second wk

OSTEOARTHRITIS
Nonpharmacologic Approaches
- Superficial heat: Hot packs, heating pads, paraffin, or hot water bottles (moist heat is better).

- Deep heat: Microwave, shortwave diathermy, or ultrasound.
- Biofeedback and transcutaneous electrical nerve stimulation.
- Exercise (especially water-based), PT, OT: Strengthening, stretching, range of motion, functional activities.
- Weight loss: Especially for low back, hip, and knee arthritis.
- Splinting: Avoid splinting for long periods of time (eg, > 6 wk) since periarticular muscle weakness and wasting may occur. Bracing (eg, neoprene sleeves over the knee) to correct malalignment is often helpful.
- Assistive devices: Cane should be used in the hand contralateral to the affected knee or hip.
- Surgical intervention (eg, debridement, meniscal repair, prosthetic joint replacement).

Pharmacologic Intervention (See **Figure 6.**)
Topical Analgesics: Liniment, capsaicin cream.
Intra-articular Injections:
- Corticosteroids: May be particularly effective if monoarticular symptoms (eg, methylprednisolone acetate, triamcinolone acetonide, and triamcinolone hexacetonide) 20–40 mg for large joints (eg, knee, ankle, shoulder), 10–20 mg for wrists and elbows, and 5–15 mg for small joints of hands and feet; often mixed with lidocaine 1% or its equivalent (in equal volume with corticosteroids) for immediate relief.
- Hyaluronan: Sodium hyaluronate (*Hyalgan*) injections weekly for 5 wk or hylan G-F 20 (*Synvisc*) 3 injections 1 wk apart for knee osteoarthritis.
Nutriceuticals: Glucosamine (500 mg 3x/d) or chondroitin (400 mg 3x/d), or both, have been effective for some patients. Combination tablets and timed-release formulations (1500 mg and 1200 mg, respectively) are available. Clinical trials in the United States are in process.
NSAIDs: Often provide pain relief but have higher rates of side effects (see **Table 49**). Misoprostol (*Cytotec*) 100–200 mg qid with food [T: 100, 200] or a proton-pump inhibitor (see **Table 32**) may be valuable prophylaxis against NSAID-induced ulcers in high-risk patients. Selective COX-2 inhibitors have lower likelihood of causing gastroduodenal ulcers than nonselective NSAIDs. All may increase INR in patients receiving warfarin.
Oral Analgesics: Eg, tramadol, other opioids (see **Table 59**).

GOUT
Definition
Urate crystal disease that may be expressed as acute gouty arthritis, usually in a single joint of foot, ankle, knee, or olecranon bursa; or chronic arthritis.

Precipitating Factors
- Alcohol, heavy ingestion
- Allopurinol, stopping or starting
- Binge eating
- Dehydration
- Diuretics
- Fasting
- Infection
- Serum uric acid levels, any change up or down
- Surgery

Figure 6. Pharmacologic Management of Osteoarthritis*

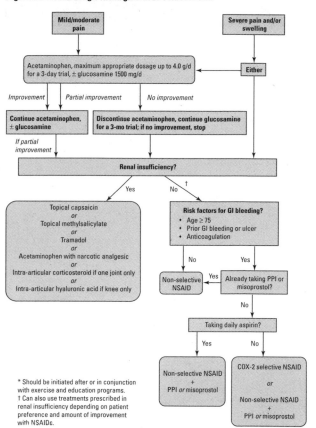

* Should be initiated after or in conjunction with exercise and education programs.
† Can also use treatments prescribed in renal insufficiency depending on patient preference and amount of improvement with NSAIDs.

Source: Adapted from original material courtesy of Catherine MacLean, MD, PhD. Reprinted with permission.

Table 49. APAP and NSAIDs

Class, Drug	Usual Dosage for Arthritis	Formulations	Comments (Metabolism, Excretion)
√APAP (*Tylenol*)	650 mg q 4–6 h	T: 80, 325, 500, 650; C: 160, 325, 500; S: elixir 120/5 mL, 160/5 mL, 167/5 mL, 325/5 mL; S: 160/5 mL, 500/15 mL; Sp: 120, 325, 600	Drug of choice for chronic musculoskeletal conditions; no anti-inflammatory properties; hepatotoxic above 4 g/d; at high doses ($\geq$ 2g/d) may increase INR in patients receiving warfarin; reduce dose 50%–75% if liver or kidney disease or if harmful or hazardous drinking (L, K)
Extended release (*Tylenol ER*)	1300 mg tid	ER: 650	
ASA	650 mg q 4–6 h	T: 81, 325, 500, 650, 975; Sp: 120, 200, 300, 600	(K)
Extended release (*Ext Release Bayer 8 Hour,* *ZORprin*)	1300 mg tid or 1600–3200 mg bid	CR: 650, 800	
Enteric-coated*	1000 mg qid	T: 81, 162, 325, 500, 650, 975	
Nonacetylated Salicylates			Do not inhibit platelet aggregation; fewer GI and renal side effects; no reaction in ASA-sensitive patients
√Choline magnesium salicylate (*Tricosal, Trilisate, CMT*)	3 g/d in 1, 2, or 3 doses	T: 500, 750, 1000; S: 500 mg/5mL	(K)
√Choline salicylate (*Arthropan*)	4.8–7.2 g/d divided	S: 870 mg/5 mL	(L, K)
√Magnesium salicylate* (eg, *Backache, Doan's, Mobigesic, Momentum*)	650 mg q 4 h, max 3600–4800/d in 3–4 divided doses; 1090 mg tid	T: 325, 377, 580; C: 467	Avoid in renal failure
√Salsalate (eg, *Disalcid, Mono-Gesic, Salflex*)	1500 mg to 4 g/d in 2 or 3 doses	T: 500, 750; C: 500	(K)
√Sodium salicylate*	325–650 mg q 4 h	T: 325, 650	

Table 49. APAP and NSAIDs (cont.)			
Class, Drug	Usual Dosage for Arthritis	Formulations	Comments (Metabolism, Excretion)
Nonselective NSAIDs			
Diclofenac (*Cataflam, Voltaren, Voltaren-XR*)	50–150 mg/d in 2 or 3 doses	T: 50, enteric coated 25, 50, 75, ER 100	(L)
√ Extended release 50 mg with 200 μg misoprostol (*Arthrotec 50*) 75 mg with 200 μg misoprostol (*Arthrotec 75*)	100 mg/d	T: 100	(L)
Diflunisal (*Dolobid*)	500–1000 mg/d in 2 doses	T: 250, 500	(K)
√Etodolac (*Lodine*)	200–400 mg tid–qid	T: 400, 500; ER 400, 500, 600;	Fewer GI side effects (L)
(*Lodine XL*)	400–1000 mg/d	C: 200, 300	
Fenoprofen (*Nalfon*)	200–600 mg tid–qid	C: 200, 300; T: 600	Higher risk of GI side effects (L)
Flurbiprofen (*Ansaid*)	200–300 mg/d in 2, 3, or 4 doses	T: 50, 100	(L)
√Ibuprofen (eg, *Advil, Motrin, Nuprin*)**	1200–3200 mg/d in 3 or 4 doses	T: 100, 200, 300, 400, 600, 800; ChT: 50, 100; S: 100 mg/5 mL	Fewer GI side effects (L)
Indomethacin (*Indochron, Indocin*)	25–50 mg bid–tid	C: 25, 50; Sp: 50; S: 25 mg/5 mL; Inj	High risk of GI side effects; increased risk of CNS side effects (L)
Extended release (*Indocin SR*)	75 mg/d or bid	C: 75	Increased risk of CNS side effects (L)
√Ketoprofen (*Actron, Orudis*)	50–75 mg tid	T: 12.5; C: 25, 50, 75	(L)
Sustained release (*Actron 200,** Oruvail*)	200 mg/d	C: 100, 150, 200	(L)
Ketorolac (*Toradol*)	10 mg q 4–6 h, 15 mg IM or IV q 6 h	T: 10; Inj	Duration of use should be limited to 5 d (K)
Meclofenamate sodium	200–400 mg/d in 3 or 4 doses	C: 50, 100	High incidence of diarrhea (L)
Mefenamic acid (*Ponstel*)	50–100 mg tid–qid 250 mg qid	T: 50, 100 T: 250	(L)
Meloxicam (*Mobic*)	7.5–15 mg/d	T: 7.5, 15	Has some COX-2 selectivity (L)
√Nabumetone (*Relafen*)	500–1000 mg bid	T: 500, 750	Fewer GI side effects (L)
√Naproxen (*Aleve,** Naprosyn*)	200–500 mg bid–tid	T: 220, 275, 375, 500; S: 125 mg/5 mL	(L)
Delayed release (*EC-Naprosyn*)	375–500 mg bid	T: 375, 500	(L)
Extended release (*Naprelan*)	750–1000 mg daily	T: 375, 500, 750	(L)

(*continues*)

Table 49. APAP and NSAIDs (cont.)			
Class, Drug	Usual Dosage for Arthritis	Formulations	Comments (Metabolism, Excretion)
Naproxen sodium (*Anaprox*)	275 mg or 550 mg bid	T: 275, 550	(L)
√Oxaprozin (*Daypro*)	1200 mg/d	C: 600	(L)
Piroxicam (*Feldene*)	10 mg/d	T: 10, 20	Can cause delirium (L)
Sulindac (*Clinoril*)	150–200 mg bid	T: 150, 200	May have higher rate of renal impairment (L)
Tolmetin (*Tolectin*)	600–1800 mg/d in 3 or 4 doses	T: 200, 600; C: 400	(L)
Selective COX-2 Inhibitors			Less GI ulceration; do not inhibit platelets; may increase INR if taking warfarin; avoid if moderate or severe hepatic insufficiency; may induce renal impairment
√Celecoxib (*Celebrex*)	100–200 mg bid	C: 100, 200	Contraindicated if allergic to sulfonamides
√Rofecoxib (*Vioxx*)	12.5–25 once daily	T: 12.5, 25, 50; S: 12.5 mg/5 mL, 25 mg/5 mL	
√Valdecoxib (*Bextra*)	10 mg once/d	T: 10, 20	

Note: √ = preferred for treating older persons.
* Also available without prescription in a lower tablet strength.
** Available without a prescription.

Evaluation of Acute Gouty Arthritis
Joint aspiration to remove crystals and microscopic examination to establish diagnosis; serum uric acid (can be normal during flare).

Management
Treatment of Acute Gouty Flare: Experts differ regarding order of choices:
• Intra-articular injections (see p 100)
• NSAIDs (see **Table 49**)
• Colchicine (more toxic in older persons; more effective if given within 24 hr of symptom onset)
  - Oral 0.5–0.6 mg (1 tablet) q 1–2 h until symptoms abate, GI toxicity occurs, or maximum dose of 6 mg/24-h period has been given.
  - IV 1–2 mg in 10–20 mL NS given over 3–5 min
    ○ may repeat the following day
    ○ contraindicated in patients who have had recent oral colchicine
    ○ avoid in patients with renal or hepatic disease
    ○ potential for severe bone marrow toxicity
• Prednisone 20–40 mg po qd until response, then rapid taper
• ACTH 75 IU SC or cosyntropin (*Cortrosyn*) 75 µg SC; may repeat daily for 3 d

Treatment of Hyperuricemia Following Acute Flare: Colchicine 0.5–0.6 mg/d for 2–4 wk before beginning any treatment in **Table 50** and continued until serum uric acid has returned to normal.

Table 50. Medications Useful in Managing Chronic Gout			
Drug	Usual Dosage	Formulations	Comments (Metabolism, Excretion)
√Allopurinol (*Zyloprim, Lopurin*)	100–200 mg qd	T: 100, 300	Do not initiate during flare; reduce dose in renal or hepatic impairment; increase dose by 100 mg every 2–4 wk to normalize serum urate level; monitor CBC; rash is common (K)
Colchicine*	0.5–0.6 mg	T: 0.5, 0.6; Inj	Follow CBC (L)
Probenecid* (*Benemid*)	500–1500 mg in 2–3 divided doses	T: 500	Adjust dose to normalize serum urate level or increase urine urate excretion; inhibits platelet function; may not be effective if renal impairment (K, L)
Sulfinpyrazone (*Anturane*)	50 mg po bid to 100 mg qid	T: 100; C: 200	Inhibits platelet function (K)

Note: √ = preferred for treating older persons.
* Probenecid (500 mg) and colchicine (0.5 mg) combinations (*ColBenemid, Col-Probenecid, Proben-C*) are available.

PSEUDOGOUT
Definition
Crystal-induced arthritis (especially affecting wrists and knees) associated with calcium pyrophosphate.

Risk Factors
- Advanced osteoarthritis
- Diabetes mellitus
- Gout
- Hemochromatosis
- Hypercalcemia
- Hyperparathyroidism
- Hypomagnesemia
- Hypophosphatemia
- Hypothyroidism
- Neuropathic joints
- Older age

Precipitating Factors
- Acute illness
- Dehydration
- Minor trauma
- Surgery

Evaluation of Acute Arthritis
Joint aspiration and microscopic examination to establish diagnosis; x-ray indicating chondrocalcinosis (best seen in wrists, knees, shoulder, symphysis pubis).

Management of Acute Flare
See **Gout** (p 100). Colchicine is less effective in pseudogout.

POLYMYALGIA RHEUMATICA, GIANT CELL (TEMPORAL) ARTERITIS
Definitions
Polymyalgia Rheumatica (PMR): Proximal limb and girdle stiffness without tenderness but with constitutional symptoms (eg, fatigue, malaise) and elevated sedimentation rate, often ≥ 100, and C-reactive protein (CRP); consider ultrasound.

Giant Cell (Temporal) Arteritis (GCA): Medium to large vessel vasculitis that presents with symptoms of PMR, headache, scalp tenderness, jaw or tongue claudication, visual disturbances, TIA or stroke, elevated sedimentation rate, and CRP.

Diagnosis and Management
- PMR is a clinical diagnosis supported by an increased sedimentation rate. Management is low-dose (eg, 5–20 mg/d) prednisone or its equivalent. Some patients with milder symptoms may respond to NSAIDs alone. Follow symptoms and CRP or sedimentation rate. Maintain therapy for at least 1 yr to prevent relapse. Consider osteoporosis prevention medication (see p 117).

- GCA is confirmed by temporal artery biopsy, but treatment should not wait for pathologic diagnosis. Begin prednisone (1.0–1.5 mg/kg/d) or its equivalent while biopsy and pathology are pending. Consider adding methotrexate 10 mg orally per wk and folate 5 mg/d, which may have a steroid-sparing effect. After 2–4 wk, begin gradual taper to lowest dose that will control symptoms and CRP or sedimentation rate. Maintain therapy for at least 1 yr to prevent relapse. Consider osteoporosis prevention medication (see p 117).

NEUROLOGIC DISORDERS

TREMORS

Table 51. Classification of Tremors				
Type	Hz	Associated Conditions	Features	Treatment
Cerebellar	3–5	Cerebellar disease	Present only during movement; ↑ with intention; ↑ amplitude as target is approached	Symptomatic management
Essential	4–12	Familial in 50% of cases	Varying amplitude; common in upper extremities, head, neck; ↑ with antigravity movements, intention, stress, medications	Long-acting propranolol or atenolol (see p 32); or primidone (*Mysoline*) 100 mg qhs start, titrate to 0.5–1.0 g/d in 3–4 divided doses [T: 50, 250; S: 250 mg/5 mL]; or gabapentin (see p 112)
Parkinson's	3–7	Parkinson's disease, parkinsonism	"Pill rolling;" present at rest; ↑ with emotional stress or when examiner calls attention to it; commonly asymmetric	See Parkinson's disease (p 110)
Physiologic	8–12	Normal	Low amplitude; ↑ with stress, anxiety, emotional upset, lack of sleep, fatigue, toxins, medications	Treatment of exacerbating factor

DIZZINESS

Table 52. Classification of Dizziness				
Primary Symptom	Features	Duration	Diagnosis	Management
Dizziness	Lightheadedness 1–30 min after standing	Seconds to minutes (E)	Orthostatic hypotension	See p 62
	Impairment in > 1 of the following: vision, vestibular function, spinal proprioception, cerebellum, lower-extremity peripheral nerves	Occurs with ambulation (C)	Multiple sensory impairments	Correct or maximize sensory deficits; PT for balance and strength training

(*continues*)

Table 52. Classification of Dizziness (cont.)

Primary Symptom	Features	Duration	Diagnosis	Management
	Unsteady gait with short steps; ↑ reflexes and/or tone	Occurs with ambulation (C)	Ischemic cerebral disease	Aspirin; modification of vascular risk factors; PT
	Provoked by head or neck movement; reduced neck range of motion	Seconds to minutes (E)	Cervical spondylosis	Behavior modification; reduce cervical spasm and inflammation
Drop attacks	Provoked by head or neck movement, reduced vertebral artery flow seen on Doppler or angiography	Seconds to minutes (E)	Postural impingement of vertebral artery	Behavior modification
Vertigo	Brought on by position change, positive Dix-Hallpike test	Seconds to minutes (E)	Benign paroxysmal positional vertigo	Epley's maneuvers to reposition crystalline debris; exercises provoking symptoms may be of help
	Acute onset, nonpositional	Days	Labyrinthitis (vestibular neuronitis)	Meclizine (see p 68)
	Low-frequency sensorineural hearing loss and tinnitus	Minutes to hours (E)	Ménière's disease	Meclizine for acute symptom relief; diuretics and/or salt restriction for prophylaxis
	Vascular disease risk factors, cranial nerve abnormalities	10 min to several hours (E)	TIAs	Aspirin; modification of vascular risk factors

Note: C = chronic; E = episodic.
Source: Data from Colledge NR, Barr-Hamilton RM, Lewis SJ, et al. Evaluation of investigations to diagnose the causes of dizziness in elderly people: a community based controlled study. *BMJ.* 1996;313(7060):788–792.

MANAGEMENT OF ACUTE STROKE
Attempt to Diagnose Cause
Examination:
- Cardiac (murmurs, arrhythmias, enlargement)
- Neurologic (serial examinations)
- Optic fundi
- Vascular (carotids and other peripheral pulses)

Tests:
• ABG	• BUN	• Creatinine	• Electrolytes
• Brain imaging (CT is adequate)	• CBC	• ECG	• ESR
	• LFTs	• Glucose	• PT/PTT/INR

Transesophageal echocardiography is preferred over transthoracic echocardiography for detection of cardiogenic emboli. Carotid duplex and transcranial Doppler studies can detect carotid and vertebrobasilar embolic sources, respectively. Magnetic resonance angiography is indicated if one is considering emergent thrombolytic therapy to reverse stroke progression within 6 h of onset of symptoms (thrombolytic therapy is of unproven benefit in older adults).

Provide Supportive Care
• Do not lower BP if SBP < 220 or if DBP < 120; higher BP should be lowered *gently*.
• Correct metabolic and hydration imbalances.
• Detect and treat coronary ischemia, HF, arrhythmias.
• Monitor and treat for hypoxia and hyperthermia.
• Monitor for depression.
• Refer to rehabilitation when medically stable.

Halt or Reverse Progression
Acute Noncardioembolic Stroke, Progressing Stroke, Crescendo TIAs, or TIA: Use ASA, 160–325 mg/d, begun within 48 h of onset. The benefit of emergent thrombolytic therapy is unproven in older adults and should be considered on a case-by-case basis. Anticoagulants are not recommended.
Cardioembolic Stroke: Begin full-dose heparin or warfarin anticoagulation 48 h after symptom onset. (See also p 17.)
Hemorrhagic Stroke: Supportive care.

STROKE PREVENTION
Risk Factor Modification
• Stop smoking
• Reduce SBP (goal < 140 mm Hg)
• Lower serum LDL (goal < 100 mg/dL)

• Start anticoagulation or antiplatelet therapy for atrial fibrillation (see p 17)

Antiplatelet Therapy for Patients With Prior TIA or Stroke
• First line is ASA 81–325 mg qd.
• Clopidogrel (*Plavix*) 75 mg qd [T: 75] if intolerant to ASA or ASA failure.
• Ticlopidine (*Ticlid*) 250 mg bid [T: 250] requires regular blood monitoring.
• Addition of dipyridamole (*Persantine*) 200–400 mg/d in 3–4 divided doses [T: 25, 50, 75] to ASA may provide additional benefit, or can be tried in cases of ASA or clopidogrel failure. A combination form of ASA (25 mg) and long-acting dipyridamole (200 mg) (*Aggrenox*) 1 tablet bid is available.
• In the absence of atrial fibrillation, warfarin therapy is no more effective than ASA in preventing strokes.

Table 53. Treatment Options for Carotid Stenosis			
Presentation	% Stenosis	Preferred Rχ	Comments
Prior TIA or stroke	≥ 70	CE	CE superior to medical therapy only if patient is reasonable surgical risk and facility has track record of low complication rate for CE (<5%)
Prior TIA or stroke	50–69	CE or MM	Serial carotid Doppler testing may identify rapidly developing plaques
Prior TIA or stroke	< 50	MM	CE of no proven benefit in this situation
Asymptomatic	≥ 80	CE or MM	CE should be considered only for the most healthy
Asymptomatic	< 80	MM	CE of no proven benefit in this situation

Note: CE = carotid endarterectomy; MM = medical management.

PARKINSON'S DISEASE
Parkinson's Disease Diagnosis Requires:
Bradykinesia, eg,
- Slowness of initiation of voluntary movements (eg, glue-footedness during gait initiation)
- Reduced speed and amplitude of repetitive movements (eg, tapping index finger and thumb together)
- Difficulty switching from one motor program to another (eg, multiple steps to turn during gait testing)

and one or more of the following:
- Muscular rigidity (eg, cogwheeling)
- 4–6 Hz resting tremor
- Impaired righting reflex (eg, retropulsed during sternal nudge)

Nonpharmacologic Management
- Patient education is essential, and support groups are often helpful; see p 203 for telephone numbers, Web sites.
- Monitor for orthostatic hypotension (see **Table 31** for management).
- Exercise program
- Surgical therapies can be considered for disabling symptoms refractory to medical therapy. Tremor can be improved by thalamotomy or thalamic stimulation (fewer side effects). Dyskinesias can be treated by pallidotomy or pallidal and subthalamic stimulation.

Table 54. Drugs for Parkinson's Disease			
Class, Drug	Initial Dosage	Formulations	Comments (Metabolism, Excretion)
Dopamine			
√ Levodopa-carbidopa* (*Sinemet*)	25/100 tid	T: 10/100, 25/100, 25/250	Mainstay of PD therapy; increase dose as needed; watch for GI side effects, orthostatic hypotension, confusion (L)
√ Sustained-release levodopa-carbidopa* (*Sinemet CR*)	1 tab bid or tid	T: 25/100, 50/200	Useful at daily dopamine requirement ≥ 300 mg; slower absorption than carbidopa-levodopa; can improve motor fluctuations (L)

Table 54. Drugs for Parkinson's Disease (cont.)			
Class, Drug	Initial Dosage	Formulations	Comments (Metabolism, Excretion)
Dopamine agonists			More CNS side effects than dopamine
Bromocriptine (*Parlodel*)	1.25 mg bid	T: 2.5; C: 5	Titrate over 3–4 wk to effective dose (15–30 mg/d); very expensive (L)
Pergolide (*Permax*)	0.05 mg qd	T: 0.05, 0.25, 1	Titrate over 3–4 wk to effective dose (2–3 mg/d in 2–3 divided doses); very expensive (K)
✓ Pramipexole* (*Mirapex*)	0.125 mg tid	T: 0.125, 0.25, 0.5, 1, 1.5	Titrate over 3–4 wk to effective dose (1.5–4.5 mg/d) (K)
✓ Ropinirole* (*Requip*)	0.25 mg tid	T: 0.25, 0.5, 1, 2, 5	Titrate over 3–4 wk to effective dose (3–16 mg/d) (L)
Catechol *O*-methyl-transferase (COMT) inhibitors			
✓ Tolcapone (*Tasmar*)	100 mg tid	T: 100, 200	Monitor LFT q 6 mo (L, K)
✓ Entacapone (*Comtan*)	200 mg with each L-dopa dose	T: 200	Adjunctive therapy with L-dopa; watch for nausea, orthostatic hypotension (L)
Anticholinergics			
Benztropine (*Cogentin*)	0.5 mg po qd	T: 0.5, 1, 2	Can cause confusion and delirium; helpful for drooling (L, K)
Trihexyphenidyl (*Artane, Trihexy*)	1 mg qd	T: 2, 5; S: 2 mg/5 mL	Same as above (L, K)
Dopamine reuptake inhibitor			
Amantadine (*Symmetrel*)	100 mg qd–bid	T: 100; C: 100; S: 50 mg/5 mL	Useful in early and late PD; watch closely for CNS side effects; do not D/C abruptly (K)
MAO B inhibitor			
Selegiline (*Carbex, Eldepryl*)	5 mg bid qam and noon	T: 5	Symptomatic benefit; not proven to be neuroprotective; expensive (L, K)

Note: ✓ = preferred for treating older persons; * = first-line therapy; PD = Parkinson's disease.

SEIZURES
Classification
- Generalized: All areas of brain affected with alteration in consciousness.
- Partial: Focal brain area affected, not necessarily with alteration in consciousness; can progress to generalized type.

Evaluation, Assessment
Initial:
- History: Neurologic disorders, trauma, drug and alcohol use
- Physical examination: General, with careful neurologic
- Routine tests: BUN, calcium, CBC, creatinine, ECG, EEG, electrolytes, glucose, head CT, LFT, magnesium
- Tests as indicated: Head MRI, lumbar puncture, oxygen saturation, urine toxic or drug screen

Common Causes:
- Advanced dementia
- CNS infection
- Drug or alcohol withdrawal
- Idiopathic causes
- Metabolic disorders
- Prior stroke (most common)
- Toxins
- Trauma
- Tumor

Management
- Treat underlying causes.
- Institute antiepileptic therapy (see **Table 55**). Virtually all antiepileptics can cause sedation and ataxia.

Table 55. Antiepileptic Therapy in Elderly Patients				
Drug	**Dosage (mg)**	**Target Blood Level (μg/mL)**	**Formulations**	**Comments (Metabolism, Excretion)**
Carbamazepine (*Tegretol*) (*Tegretol XR*)	200–600 bid	4–12	T: 200; ChT: 100; S: 100/5 mL T: 100, 200, 400; C: CR 200, 300	Many drug interactions; mood stabilizer; may cause SIADH, thrombocytopenia, leukopenia (L, K)
Gabapentin (*Neurontin*)	300–600 tid	NA	C: 100, 300, 400; T: 600, 800; S: 250/5 mL	Used as adjunct to other agents; adjust dose on basis of CrCl (K)
Lamotrigine (*Lamictal*)	100–300 bid	2–4	T: 25, 100, 150, 200; ChT: 2, 5, 25	Prolongs PR interval; when used with valproic acid, begin at 25 mg qd, titrate to 25–100 mg bid (L, K)
Levetiracetam (*Keppra*)	500–1500 q 12 h	NA	T: 250, 500, 750	Reduce dose in renal impairment: CrCl 30–50: 250–750 q 12 h CrCl 10–30: 250–750 q 12 h CrCl < 10: 500–1000 q 24 h
Oxcarbazepine (*Trileptal*)	300–1200 bid	NA	T: 150, 300, 600; ChT: 2, 5, 25; S: 300/5 mL	Can cause hyponatremia (L)
Phenobarbital (*Luminal*)	30–60 bid–tid	20–40	T: 15, 16, 30, 32, 60, 100; S: 20/5 mL	Many drug interactions; not recommended for use in elderly patients (L)
Phenytoin (*Dilantin*)	200–300 qd	5–20*	C: 30, 100; ChT: 50; S: 125/5 mL	Many drug interactions; exhibits nonlinear pharmacokinetics (L)
Tiagabine (*Gabitril Filmtabs*)	2–12 bid–tid	NA	T: 2, 4, 12, 16, 20	Side-effect profile in elderly patients less well described (L)
Topiramate (*Topamax*)	25–100 qd–bid	NA	T: 25, 100, 200; C, sprinkle: 15, 25	May affect cognitive functioning at high doses (L, K)

Table 55. Antiepileptic Therapy in Elderly Patients (cont.)				
Drug	Dosage (mg)	Target Blood Level (μg/mL)	Formulations	Comments (Metabolism, Excretion)
Valproic acid (*Depacon, Depakene, Depakote*)	250–750 bid–tid	50–100	T: ER 125, 250, 500; C: 125, 250; S: 250/5 mL	Can cause weight gain; several drug interactions; mood stabilizer; follow LFTs and platelets; SR preparation (*Depakote ER*) also available [T: 500] (L)

Note: NA = not available.

* Phenytoin is extensively bound to plasma albumin. In cases of hypoalbuminemia or marked renal insufficiency, calculate adjusted phenytoin concentration (C):

$$C_{adjusted} = \frac{C_{observed} \; (\mu g/mL)}{0.2 \times albumin \, (g/dL) + 0.1}$$

If creatinine clearance < 10 mL/min, use:

$$C_{adjusted} = \frac{C_{observed} \; (\mu g/mL)}{0.1 \times albumin \, (g/dL) + 0.1}$$

Obtaining a free phenytoin level is an alternate method for monitoring phenytoin in cases of hypoalbuminemia or marked renal insufficiency.

APHASIA

Table 56. Aphasias In Which Repetition Is Impaired				
Type	Fluency	Auditory Comprehension	Associated Neurologic Deficits	Comments
Broca's	−	+	Right hemiparesis	Patient aware of deficit; high rate of associated depression; message board helpful for communication
Wernicke's	+	−	Often none	Patient frequently unaware of deficit; speech content usually unintelligible; therapy often focuses on visually based communication
Conduction	+	+	Occasional right facial weakness	Patient usually aware of the deficit; speech content usually intelligible
Global	−	−	Right hemiplegia with right field cut	Most commonly due to left middle cerebral artery thrombosis, which, if this is the cause, carries a poor prognosis for meaningful speech recovery

Note: + = present; − = absent

Figure 7. Diagnosis of Peripheral Neuropathy

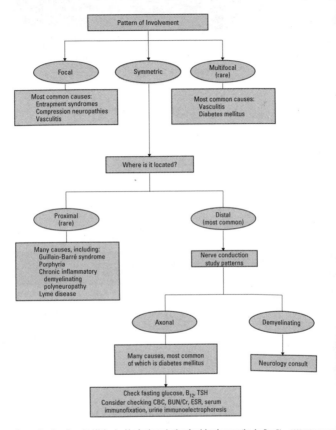

Source: Data from Poncelet AN. An algorithm for the evaluation of peripheral neuropathy. *Am Fam Phys.* 1998;57(4):755–764.

PERIPHERAL NEUROPATHY

Diagnosis
See **Figure 7**.

Treatment
Prevention of Complications:
- Protect distal extremities from trauma—appropriate shoe size, daily foot inspections, good skin care, avoidance of barefoot walking.
- Maintain tight glycemic control in diabetic neuropathy.

Treatment of Painful Neuropathy: Start at low dose, increase as needed and tolerated:
- Nortriptyline (*Aventyl, Pamelor*) 10–100 mg qhs [T: 10, 25, 50, 75]; desipramine (*Norpramin*) 10–75 mg qam [T: 10, 25, 50, 75]
- Gabapentin (*Neurontin*) can begin 100–200 mg qhs but may need up to 100–600 mg tid [C: 100, 300, 400; T: 600, 800; S: 250/5 mL]
- Other oral agents that may be effective include:
  - Carbamazepine: (*Tegretol*) 200–400 mg tid [T: 200; ChT: 100; S: 100 mg/5 mL]; (*Tegretol XR*) 200 mg bid [T: 100, 200, 400; C: CR 200, 300]
  - SSRIs (**Table 60**) have not been shown to be as effective as tricyclics
  - Lamotrigine (*Lamictal*, see **Table 55**) 400–600 mg/d
  - Opioids (**Table 59**); watch for side effects of itching, mood changes, weakness, confusion
  - Tramadol (*Ultram*, see **Table 59**) 200–400 mg/d
- Topical agents that may be effective include:
  - Capsaicin cream (eg, *Zostrix*) 0.075% applied tid–qid [0.025%, 0.075%]
  - Transcutaneous electrical nerve stimulation
  - Lidocaine 5% patches (*Lidoderm*) 1–3 patches covering the affected area up to 12 h/d [700 mg patch]

OSTEOPOROSIS

COMMONLY USED DEFINITIONS
- Established osteoporosis: occurrence of a minimal trauma fracture of any bone (WHO)
- Osteoporosis: a skeletal disorder characterized by compromised bone strength (bone density and bone quality) predisposing to an increased risk of fracture: NIH Consensus Development Panel. Osteoporosis prevention, diagnosis, and therapy. *JAMA* 2001; 285 (6):785–795.
- Osteoporosis: BMD 2.5 SD or more below that of younger normal individuals (T score) (WHO). Some experts prefer to use Z score, which compares an individual with a population adjusted for age, sex, and race. For each SD decrement in BMD, hip fracture risk increases about 2-fold; for each SD increment in BMD, hip fracture risk is about halved.

RISK FACTORS FOR OSTEOPOROTIC FRACTURE
- Previous fracture as adult
- Dementia
- Depression
- Low calcium intake
- Impaired vision
- Low physical activity
- Fracture in 1st-degree relative
- Frailty
- Alcoholism
- Female sex
- Weight < 127 lb if female
- Cigarette smoking
- Early menopause (< 45 yr)
- Recurrent falls

TOXINS AND MEDICATIONS THAT CAN CAUSE OR AGGRAVATE OSTEOPOROSIS
- Alcohol (> 2 drinks/d)
- Anticonvulsants
- Corticosteroids
- Heparin
- Lithium
- Phenytoin
- Smoking
- Thyroxine (if overreplaced or in suppressive doses)

EVALUATION
Some experts recommend excluding secondary causes (serum PTH, TSH, calcium, phosphorus, albumin, alkaline phosphatase, bioavailable testosterone in men, renal and liver function tests, CBC, UA, electrolytes, protein electrophoresis). Less consensus on vitamin D levels, 24-h urinary calcium excretion, cortisol, antibodies associated with gluten-enteropathy; BMD test only if results could influence treatment or to establish baseline (see screening p 134). The value of monitoring BMD in persons already receiving treatment is unproven.

MANAGEMENT
Universal Recommendations
- Calcium 1200 mg/d*
- Vitamin D 400–800 IU
- Avoid tobacco
- Weight-bearing exercise
- Falls prevention
- No more than moderate alcohol use

*For most patients, calcium carbonate is sufficient and least expensive. For patients on proton-pump inhibitors (see **Table 32**) or who have achlorhydria, calcium citrate should be used.

Pharmacologic Prevention
- Most organizations have recommended initiating pharmacologic management in women with BMD T scores below −2 in the absence of risk factors and in women with T scores below −1.5 if other risk factors are present.
- Regimens:
  - Alendronate (*Fosamax*) 5 mg/d or 35 mg/wk [T: 5, 10, 35, 40, 70] (must be taken fasting with water; patient must remain upright and npo for at least 30 min after taking; relatively contraindicated in GERD) *or*
  - Risedronate (*Actonel*) 35 mg/wk or 5 mg/d [T: 5, 30, 35] (must be taken fasting or at least 2 h after evening meal; patient must remain upright and npo for 30 min after taking) *or*
  - Raloxifene (*Evista*) 60 mg/d [T: 60] *or*
  - Estrogen without progesterone (only women with hysterectomy) (see **Table 83** for dosing).

Nonpharmacologic Treatment
Vertebroplasty (injection of bone cement into a collapsed vertebra) or kyphoplasty (inflation of a balloon tamp before cement injection) has improved pain and function acutely in case studies and nonrandomized controlled studies; long-term benefits for pain, function, and vertebral height are uncertain.

Pharmacologic Treatment for Those with Prior Osteoporotic Fractures
- Alendronate (*Fosamax*) 10 mg/d or 70 mg/wk [T: 5, 10, 35, 40, 70] (must be taken fasting with water; patient must remain upright and npo for at least 30 min after taking; relatively contraindicated in GERD) *or*
- Risedronate (*Actonel*) 35 mg/wk or 5 mg/d [T: 5, 30, 35] (must be taken fasting or at least 2 h after evening meal; patient must remain upright and npo for 30 min after taking) *or*
- Raloxifene (*Evista*) 60 mg/d [T: 60] *or*
- Calcitonin (*Calcimar, Cibacalcin, Miacalcin, Osteocalcin, Salmonine*) 100 IU/d SC [Inj: human (*Cibacalcin*) 0.5 mg/vial; salmon 200 units/mL) or 200 IU (*Miacalcin*) [200 units/activation] (intranasally, alternate nostrils every other day). May also be helpful for analgesic effect in patients with acute vertebral fracture (see also p 98) *or*
- Estrogen without progesterone (only women with hysterectomy) (see **Table 83** for dosing).
- Teriparatide (*Forteo*) 20 μg/d for up to 24 mo [Inj 3 mL, 28-dose disposable pen device] for high-risk patients; contraindicated in patients with Paget's disease or prior skeletal radiation therapy (L, K).

Table 57. Bone Outcomes and Level of Evidence* of Drugs for Osteoporosis

Drug	Spine BMD and Fracture	Hip BMD	Hip Fracture	All Nonspinal Fractures
Estrogen**	improved–R	improved–R	reduced–R	no effect–R
Raloxifene	improved–R	improved–R	no data	no effect–R
Alendronate	improved–R	improved–R	reduced–R	reduced–R
Risedronate	improved–R	improved–R	reduced–R	reduced–R
Calcitonin (nasal)	improved–R	no effect–R	no effect–R	no effect–R
Teriparatide	improved–R	improved–R	no data	reduced–R

* The populations studied, sample sizes of individual studies, and duration of follow-up vary considerably; hence, this summary must be interpreted cautiously. Moreover, several randomized clinical trials are currently in progress and new findings may appear.
** The least expensive of the drugs listed.
Note: R = randomized clinical trial.

Table 58. Effects on Other Outcomes, Level of Evidence,* and Risks of Drugs for Osteoporosis

Drug	CHD Risk Factors	CHD Prevention	CHD Treatment	Breast Cancer	Deep-Vein Thrombosis	Other
Estrogen	improved–R	↑ risk–R	no effect–R	↑ risk–R	↑ risk–R	↑ vaginal bleeding, stroke, PE ↓ colorectal cancer–R
Raloxifene	improved–R	↓ risk–R**	↓ risk–R	↓ risk–R	↑ risk–R	↑ hot flushes–R
Alendronate	no data	no data	no data	no data	no data	esophagitis
Risedronate	no data	no data	no data	no data	no data	
Calcitonin (nasal)	no data	no data	no data	no data	no data	rhinitis in 10%–12%

* The populations studied, sample sizes of individual studies, and duration of follow-up vary considerably; hence, this summary must be interpreted cautiously. Moreover, several randomized clinical trials are currently in progress and new findings may appear.
** Reduced risk demonstrated for high-risk women only.
Note: CHD = coronary heart disease; R = randomized clinical trial.

DEFINITION
An unpleasant sensory and emotional experience associated with actual or potential tissue damage (International Association for Study of Pain taxonomy)

Acute Pain
Distinct onset, usually evident pathology, short duration; common causes: post-surgical pain, trauma

Persistent Pain
Persistent (lasting longer than expected trajectory), often associated with functional and psychologic impairment, can fluctuate in character and intensity over time; common causes: arthritis, cancer, claudication, leg cramps, neuropathy, radiculopathy, low back pain, myofascial pain syndromes

EVALUATION
Key Points, Approach
- Assume patient's report is the most reliable evidence of pain intensity.
- Assess for pain on each presentation (older adults may be reluctant to report pain).
- Use synonyms for pain (eg, burning, aching, soreness, discomfort).
- Use a standard pain scale (see p 191); adapt for sensory impairments (eg, large print, written versus spoken).
- Assess cognitively impaired patients by:
  - Using simple tools or questions with yes/no answers.
  - Noting increased vocalizations (eg, moaning, groaning, crying).
  - Observing behaviors (eg, grimacing, irritability, failure to move an extremity, guarding).
  - Asking caregiver about recent changes in function, gait, behavior patterns, mood.
- Use a screening approach to recognize potential pain problems in nonverbal, cognitively impaired elders (see **Figure 8**).
- Reassess regularly for improvement, deterioration, complications; keep log.
- Refer for comprehensive multidisciplinary evaluation for complex pain problem.

History and Physical
- Focus on a complete examination of pain source.
- Distinguish new illness from chronic condition.
- Analgesic history: effectiveness and side effects, current and previous prescription drugs, OTC drugs, "natural" remedies.
- Laboratory and diagnostic tests: to establish etiologic diagnosis.

Characteristics of Pain Complaint
Provocative (aggravating) and **P**alliative (relieving) factors
Quality (eg, burning, stabbing, dull, throbbing)
Region
Severity (eg, scale of 0 for no pain to 10 for worst pain possible; see p 191)
Timing (eg, when pain occurs, frequency and duration)

Figure 8. Pain Assessment in Elders with Severe Cognitive Impairment

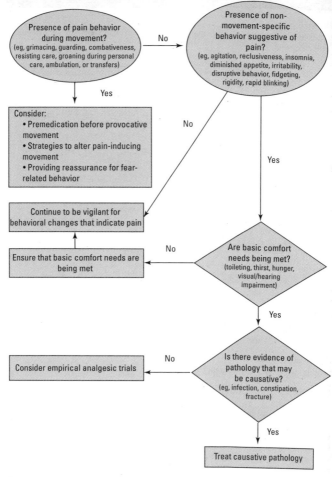

Sources: Adapted with permission from American Geriatrics Society. The management of persistent pain in older persons. *J Amer Geriatr Soc* 2002; 50 (Suppl S205–S224): and Weiner D, Herr K, Rudy T, eds. Persistent Pain in Older Adults: An Interdisciplinary Guide for Treatment, 2002, Copyright Springer Publishing Company, Inc., New York 10012.

Psychosocial Assessment

Depression (see p 185 for screen), anxiety, mental status (see p 183 for screen). Enabling behaviors by others (eg, oversolicitousness, co-dependency, reinforcing debility)

Functional Assessment

ADLs, impact on activities (see pp 183–185 for screens) and quality of life.

Brief Pain Inventory

Use for comprehensive assessment of pain and its impact (see p 193).

PAIN MANAGEMENT

Acute Pain and Short-Term Management

- Use fixed schedule of APAP, NSAIDs (consider nonselective versus COX-2 inhibitors depending on risk factors and co-morbidities, see **Figure 6**), or opioids.
- For severe pain, consider patient-controlled analgesic pump.
- Include nonpharmacologic strategies (eg, relaxation, heat or cold).

Persistent Pain

- Use multidisciplinary assessment and treatment.
- Educate patient for self-management and coping.
- Combine drug and nondrug strategies.
- Anticipate and attend to depression and anxiety.
- Provide instruction in self-conditioning, strengthening, flexibility, stretching (all per patient's ability).

Nonpharmacologic Treatment

- Educate patient and caregiver.
- Emphasize self-administered therapies (eg, heat, cold, massage, liniments and topical agents).
- Prescribe exercise, especially for persistent pain (see p 136).
- Add therapy conducted by professionals (eg, distraction, relaxation techniques, music therapy, coping skills, biofeedback, imagery, hypnosis) as needed.
- When appropriate, obtain:
  - Rehabilitation medicine consult (OT, PT) for mechanical devices to minimize pain and facilitate activity (eg, splints), transcutaneous electrical nerve stimulation, range-of-motion and ADL programs.
  - Psychiatric pain management consult for somatization or hysteria, management of withdrawal.
  - Anesthesia pain management consult for possible interventional therapy (eg, neuroaxial analgesia, injection therapy, neuromodulation) when more conservative approaches are ineffective.

Pharmacologic Treatment
Selection of Agent(s):

- Base initial choice of analgesic on the severity and type of pain (see Osteoarthritis, **Figure 6**):
  - Consider nonopioids for mild pain (rating 1–3) (see **Table 49**).
  - Consider low-dose combination agents (see **Table 59**) for mild to moderate pain (rating 4–6) (eg, oxycodone, hydrocodone, tramadol with APAP).

- Consider potent and titratable mu opioid agonists (see **Table 59**) for more severe pain (rating 7–10) (eg, morphine, hydromorphone, oxycodone, fentanyl).
- Consider adjuvant drugs (see **Table 60**) alone or in conjunction with opioids or nonopioids for neuropathic pain and other selected chronic conditions.
- Select lowest side-effect profile agents.
• Select least invasive route (usually oral) and fast-onset, short-acting analgesics for episodic or breakthrough pain.
• Use long-acting or sustained-release analgesics for continuous pain.
• Avoid long-term, nonselective NSAID use for chronic conditions.
• Consider COX-2 inhibitors for patients who would benefit from anti-inflammatory drug therapy on a continuous, long-term basis.
• Consider fixed-dose combinations (eg, APAP and hydrocodone or tramadol) for mild to moderate pain; do not exceed maximum dose for nonopioid.
• Avoid using multiple opioids or nonopioids when possible.
• Drugs with long half-life or depot effects (eg, methadone, levorphanol, transdermal fentanyl) need to be used and titrated cautiously, with close supervision of effects; duration of effect may exceed usual dose intervals because of reductions in metabolism and clearance.

Adjustment of Dosage:
• Begin with lowest dose possible, increasing slowly.
• Titrate dose on basis of persistent need for and use of medications for breakthrough pain. If using 3 or more doses of breakthrough pain medication per day, consider increased dose of sustained-release medication.
• Dose to therapeutic ceiling of nonopioid or NSAID if side effects permit.
• Increase opioid dose until pain relief achieved or side effects unmanageable before changing drugs (there is no maximum dose or analgesic ceiling with opioids).
• Use morphine equivalents as a common denominator for all dose conversions to avoid errors.
• When changing opioids, decrease equianalgesic dose by 25%–50% because of incomplete tolerance.
• Administer around-the-clock for continuous pain.
• Reassess, re-examine, and readjust therapy frequently until pain is relieved.

Management of Side Effects:
• Anticipate, prevent, and vigorously treat side effects; expect older patients to be more sensitive to side effects.
• Begin prophylactic laxative, osmotic, or stimulant when initiating opioid therapy (see **Table 34**); if patient taking sufficient fluids, cautiously increase fiber or psyllium; titrate laxative dose up with opiate dose. (See also p 66 stepped approach.)
• Monitor for sedation, delirium, urinary retention, constipation, respiratory depression, and nausea; tolerance develops to mild sedation, nausea, and impaired cognitive function.
• On long-term NSAID use, monitor periodically for GI blood loss, renal insufficiency, and other drug-drug and drug-disease interactions.
• Avoid the following drugs: carisoprodol, chlorzoxazone, cyclobenzaprine, indomethacin, meperidine, metaxalone, methocarbamol, nalbuphine, pentazocine, propoxyphene (see also p 200 for CMS criteria regarding inappropriate drug use).

Table 59. Opioid Analgesic Drugs				
Class, Drug	MS Equiv* (Route)	Starting Oral Dosage in Opioid-Naïve Patients	Formulations	Indication for Pain**
Short-Acting				
Codeine	200 mg (po)	15 mg q 4–6 h	T: 15, 30, 60; S: 15/ 5 mL; Inj	A
Codeine & APAP†	200 mg (po)	1–2 15/325 tabs q 4–6 h; if 1 tab used, add 325 mg APAP	T: 15/325, 30/325, 60/325, 30/500, 30/650, 7.5/300, 15/300, 30/300, 60/300; S: 12/120/5 mL	A
Hydrocodone & APAP† (eg, *Lorcet, Lortab, Vicodin*)	30 mg	5–10 mg q 4–6 h	T: 10/325, 5/400, 7.5/400, 10/400, 2.5/500, 5/500, 7.5/500, 10/500, 7.5/500, 7.5/750, 10/650, 10/660; C: 5/500; S: 2.5/167/ 5 mL (contains 7% alcohol)	A
Hydrocodone & ASA (eg, *Lortab ASA*)	30 mg	5/500	T: 5/500	A
Hydrocodone & ibuprofen (eg, *Vicoprofen*)	30 mg	7.5/200	T: 7.5/200	A
Oxycodone (*Oxy IR, Roxicodone*)	20–30 mg (po)	5 mg q 3–4 h	T: 5, 15, 30; C: 5; S: 5 mg/mL, 20 mg/mL	A
Oxycodone & APAP† (*Percocet, Tylox*)	20 mg (po)	2.5–5 mg oxycodone q 6 h	T: 2.5/325, 5/325, 5/500, 7.5/325, 7.5/500, 10/325, 10/650; C: 5/500; S: 5/325/5 mL	A
Oxycodone & ASA (*Percodan*)	20 mg (po)	2.25–4.5 mg oxycodone q 6 h	T: 2.25/325, 4.5/325	A
Morphine (*MSIR, Astramorph PF, Duramorph, Infumorph, Roxanol, OMS Concentrate, MS/L, RMS, MS/S*)	30 mg (po), 10 mg (IV, IM, SC)	5 mg (po), 1–2 mg (IV) q 4–6 h	C: 15, 30; soluble T: 15, 30; S: 10 mg/5 mL, 20 mg/5 mL, 100 mg/5 mL, 4 mg/mL, 20 mg/mL; Sp: 5, 10, 20, 30; Inj	B
Hydromorphone (*Dilaudid, Hydrostat*)	7.5 mg (po), 1.5 mg (IV, IM, SC), 6 mg (rectal)	2 mg q 3–4 h	T: 2, 4, 8; S: 5 mg/5 mL; Sp: 3; Inj	B

(*continues*)

Class, Drug	MS Equiv* (Route)	Starting Oral Dosage in Opioid-Naïve Patients	Formulations	Indication for Pain**
Oxymorphone (*Numorphan*)	1 mg (IV, IM, SC), 10 mg (rectal)	0.5 mg IM, IV, SC q 4–6 h	Sp: 5; Inj	B
Fentanyl (*Actiq*)	NA	suck on 200 μg loz over 15 min, effect begins within 10 min	loz on a stick: 200, 400, 600, 800, 1200, 1600 μg	B
Tramadol (*Ultram*)	150–300 mg	25–50 mg q 4–6 h; not > 300 for age 75+	T: 50	B
Tramadol & APAP† (*Ultracet*)	37.5/325 mg	2 tabs po q 4–6 h pain; max 8 tabs/d‡	T: 37.5/325	B
Long-Acting				
ER Morphine (*MS Contin, Kadian, Avinza*)	30 mg (po) *MS Contin* and *Kadian*, 60 mg (po) *Avinza*	20–30 mg q 24 h, 15 mg q 12 h (*MS Contin* CR and XR tabs), 20 mg q 24 h (*Kadian* SR caps), 30 mg q 24 h (*Avinza* caps)	T: CR 15, 30, 60, 100, 200, XR 15, 30, 60; C: SR 5, 20, 30, 60, 100; C: 30, 60, 90, 120	B
ER Oxycodone (*OxyContin*)	20–30 mg (po)	20 mg q 24 h, 10 mg q 12 h	T: CR 10, 20, 40, 80, 160	B
Transdermal fentanyl§ (*Duragesic*)	NA (see package insert)	25 μg/h or higher (if able to tolerate 50 mg oral morphine equiv/ 24 h)	25 μg/h (10 cm²), 50 μg/h (20 cm²), 75 μg/h (30 cm²), 100 μg/h (40 cm²)	B

* MS Equiv = morphine sulphate (MS) equivalent dose: morphine equivalency = dose of opioid equivalent to 10 mg of parenteral morphine or 30 mg of oral morphine with chronic dosing. The parenteral:oral ratio is greater (1:6) during acute dosing, ie, 10 mg IM MS = 60 mg po MS. NA = not applicable.

** A = mild to moderate pain; B = moderate to severe pain.

† Caution: total APAP dose should not exceed 4 g/d.

‡ Treatment not to exceed 5 d; if CrCl < 30 mL/min, max is 2 tab q 12 h, not to exceed 5 d.

§ Caution: Active ingredient accumulates in subcutaneous fat, thus duration of action may be >17 h. Do not use in opioid-naïve patients. Do not apply heat to patch. Not recommended for treatment of acute pain.

Table 60. Adjuvant Drugs for Pain Relief in Elderly Patients			
Class, Drug	**Formulations**	**Starting Dosage**	**Comments**
Anticonvulsants (see **Table 55** and p 115)			If one does not work, try another
Antidepressants (see **Table 25**)			Use low-dose desipramine or nortryptiline; data on SSRIs lacking
Corticosteroids (see **Table 28**)			Low-dose medical management may be helpful in inflammatory conditions
Counterirritants			
√ Camphor-menthol-phenol (*Sarna*)*	lot: camphor 5%, menthol 5%, phenol 5%	prn	May be effective for arthritic pain, but effect limited when pain affects multiple joints; can cause skin injury, especially if used with heat or occlusive dressing
√ Camphor and phenol (*Campho-Phenique*)*	S: camphor 5%, phenol 4.7%	prn	
√ Methylsalicylate and menthol (*Ben-Gay* oint,* *Icy Hot* crm*)	methylsalicylate 18.3%, menthol 16%	3–4 × / d	Apply to affected area
(*Ben-Gay* extra strength crm*)	methylsalicylate 30%, menthol 10%	3–4 × / d	Apply to affected area
√ Trolamine salicylate (*Aspercreme* rub*)	trolamine salicylate 10%	≤ 4 × / d	Apply to affected area
Other agents			
Baclofen (*Lioresal*)	T: 10, 20; Inj	2.5–5 mg bid–tid	Probably increased sensitivity and decreased clearance; monitor for weakness, urinary dysfunction; avoid abrupt discontinuation because of CNS irritability
√ Capsaicin (eg, *Capsin, Capzasin, No Pain-HP, R-Gel, Zostrix*)	crm, lot, gel, roll-on: 0.025%, 0.075%	3–4 × / d	Renders skin and joints insensitive by depleting and preventing reaccumulation of substance P in peripheral sensory neurons; may cause burning sensation; instruct patient to wash hands after application to prevent eye contact; do not apply to open or broken skin

√ = preferred for treating older persons.
* Available OTC.
Note: Various adjuvant classes are useful for the treatment of neuropathic pain. TCAs are often helpful for migraine or tension headaches and arthritic conditions. Baclofen is particularly useful for muscle-related problems, such as spasms.

PALLIATIVE AND END-OF-LIFE CARE

DEFINITION
"Palliative care is an approach to care which improves quality of life of patients and their families facing life-threatening illnesses, through the prevention and relief of suffering by means of early identification and impeccable assessment and treatment of pain and other problems, physical, psychosocial, and spiritual." (WHO, 2002)

PRINCIPLES
- Support, educate, and treat both patient and family.
- Address physical, psychologic, social, and spiritual needs.
- Use multidisciplinary team (physicians, nurses, social workers, chaplain, pharmacist, physical and occupational therapists, dietitian, family and caregivers, volunteers).
- Focus on symptom management, comfort, meeting goals, completion of "life business," healing relationships, and bereavement.
- Make care available 24 h/d, 7 d/wk.
- Offer bereavement support.
- Provide therapeutic environment (palliation can be given in any location).
- Advocate comprehensive palliative care for all dying patients.

QUALITY OF LIFE
Ways to help patient and family enhance quality of life at the end of life:
- Communicate, listen
- Teach stress management, coping
- Use all available resources
- Support decision making
- Encourage conflict resolution
- Help complete unfinished business
- Urge focus on non-illness-related affairs
- Urge a focus on one day at a time
- Help anticipate grief, losses
- Help focus on attainable goals
- Encourage spiritual practices
- Promote physical, psychologic comfort

END-OF-LIFE DECISIONS
Follow principles involved in informed decision making (see **Figure 2**).
Hospice Referral
- Patients, families, or other health care provides can refer, but a physician's order is required for admission to a hospice program.
- Referral is appropriate when curative treatment is no longer indicated (ie, ineffective, too burdensome side effects) and life is limited to months.
- Hospice must be accepted by the patient or family, or both, and can be rescinded at any time.
- Hospice provides palliative medications, durable medical supplies and equipment, team member visits as needed and desired by patient and family (physician, nurses, home health aide, social worker, chaplain) and volunteer services.
- Optimal hospice care requires adequate time in the program; referral when death is imminent does not take full advantage of hospice care.
- Hospice care is usually delivered in patient's home, but it can be delivered in a nursing home or residential care facility (long-term care, assisted living) or in an inpatient

setting (hospice-specific or contracted facility) if acuity or social circumstances warrant.

Advance Directives
Designed to respect patient's autonomy and determine his/her wishes about future life-sustaining medical treatment if unable to indicate wishes.

Oral Statements
- Conversations with relatives, friends, clinicians are most common form; should be thoroughly documented in medical record for later reference.
- Properly verified oral statements carry same ethical and legal weight as those recorded in writing.

Instructional Advance Directives (DNR Orders, Living Wills)
- Written instructions regarding the initiation, continuation, withholding, or withdrawal of particular forms of life-sustaining medical treatment.
- May be revoked or altered at any time by the patient.
- Clinicians who comply with such directives are provided legal immunity for such actions.

Durable Power of Attorney for Health Care or Health Care Proxy
A written document that enables a capable person to appoint someone else to make future medical treatment choices for him or her in the event of decisional incapacity (see **Figure 2**).

Key Interventions, Treatment Decisions to Include in Advance Directives:
- Resuscitation procedures
- Mechanical respiration
- Chemotherapy, radiation therapy
- Dialysis
- Simple diagnostic tests
- Pain control
- Blood products, transfusions
- Intentional deep sedation

Withholding or Withdrawing Therapy
- There is no ethical or legal difference between withholding an intervention (not starting it) and withdrawing life-sustaining medical treatment (stopping it after it has been started).
- Beginning a treatment does not preclude stopping it later; a time-limited trial may be appropriate.
- Palliative care should not be limited, even if life-sustaining treatments are withdrawn or withheld.
- Decisions on artificial feeding should be based on the same criteria applied to ventilators and other medical treatment.

Euthanasia
- Active euthanasia: direct intervention, such as lethal injection, intended to hasten a patient's death; a criminal act of homicide.
- Passive euthanasia: withdrawal or withholding of unwanted or unduly burdensome life-sustaining treatment; appropriate in certain circumstances.
- Assisted suicide: the patient's intentional, willful ending of his/her own life with the assistance of another; a criminal offense in most states.

MANAGEMENT OF COMMON END-OF-LIFE SYMPTOMS

Pain

- The most distressing symptom for patients and caregivers.
- If intent is to relieve suffering, the risk that sufficient medication will produce an unintended effect (hastening death) is morally acceptable.
- Primary goal: to alleviate suffering at end of life. See Pain (p 119) for assessment and interventions.
- Alternate routes may be needed, eg, transdermal, transmucosal, rectal, vaginal, topical, epidural, and intrathecal.
- Recommend expert pain management consult if pain not adequately relieved with standard analgesic guidelines and interventions.
- Additional treatment may include:
  - radionuclides and bisphosphonates (for metastatic bone pain).
  - treatments (eg, radiotherapy, chemotherapy) directed at source of pain.
- Pain crisis: Sedation at end of life for intractable pain and suffering is an important option to discuss with patients. Ketamine (*Ketalar*) 0.1 mg/kg IV bolus. Repeat as needed q 5 min. Follow with infusion of 0.015 mg/kg/min IV (SC if IV access not available at 0.3–0.5 mg/kg). Decrease opioid dose by 50%. Benzodiazepine may be useful. Observe for problems with increased secretions and treat (see section on excessive secretions, p 130).

Weakness, Fatigue

Nonpharmacologic:

- Modify environment to decrease energy expenditure (eg, placement of phone, bedside commode, and drinks).
- Adjust room temperature to patient's comfort.
- Teach energy-conserving techniques (eg, reordering tasks—eating first, resting, then bathing).
- Modify daily procedures (eg, sitting while showering, not standing).

Pharmacologic:

- Treat remediable causes such as pain, medication toxicity, insomnia, anemia, and depression.
- Consider psychostimulants (eg, dextroamphetamine [*Dexedrine*] 2.5 mg po qam or bid *or* methylphenidate [*Ritalin*] 5–10 mg po qam or bid); monitor for signs of psychosis, agitation, or sleep disturbance.

Dysphagia

Nonpharmacologic:

- Feed small, frequent amounts of pureed or soft foods.
- Avoid spicy, salty, acidic, sticky, and extremely hot or cold foods.
- Keep head of bed elevated for 30 min after eating.
- Instruct patient to wear dentures and to chew thoroughly.
- Use suction machine when necessary.

Pharmacologic:

- For painful mucositis: 1:2:8 mixture of diphenhydramine elixir: lidocaine [2%–4%]: magnesium-aluminum hydroxide (eg, *Maalox*) as a swish-and-swallow suspension before meals.

- For candidiasis: clotrimazole 10 mg troches, 5 doses/d, *or* fluconazole 150 mg po followed by 100 mg po qd × 5 d.
- For severe halitosis: antimicrobial mouthwash; fastidious oral and dental care; treat putative respiratory tract infection with broad-spectrum antibiotics.

Dyspnea
Nonpharmacologic:
- Teach positions to facilitate breathing, elevate head of bed.
- Teach relaxation techniques.
- Eliminate smoke and allergens.
- Assure brisk air circulation (facial breeze) with a room fan; oxygen is indicated only for symptomatic hypoxemia (ie, $SaO_2 < 90\%$ with pulse oximetry).

Pharmacologic:
- Opioids: oral morphine conc (20 mg/mL): 1/4 to 1/2 mL sl/po; repeat in 10–15 min prn); nebulized morphine 2.5 mg in 2–4 cc NS *or* fentanyl 25–50 μg in 2–4 cc NS; *or* IV morphine 1 mg or equivalent opioid q 5–10 min.
- Bronchodilators (see **Table 71**).
- Diuretics, if evidence of volume overload (see **Table 18**).
- Anxiolytics (eg, lorazepam po/sl/SC 0.5–2 mg q 2–4 h or prn); titrate slowly to effect.

Constipation
Most common cause: side effects of opioids, medications with anticholinergic side-effects (see **Table 34**). Use stimulant or osmotic laxative.

Bowel Obstruction
Indications for Radiographic Evaluation:
- To differentiate constipation and mechanical obstruction
- To confirm the obstruction, determine site and nature if surgery is being considered

Nonpharmacologic Management:
- Nasogastric intubation: only if surgery is being considered, for high-level obstructions, and poor response to pharmacotherapy
- Percutaneous venting gastrostomy: for high-level obstructions and profuse vomiting not responsive to antiemetics
- Palliative surgery
- Hydration: IV or hypodermoclysis

Pharmacologic Management (aimed at specific symptoms):
- Nausea and vomiting: haloperidol (*Haldol*) po, IM 0.5–5 mg ($\leq$ 10 mg) q 4–8 h prn; ondansetron (*Zofran*) IV (over 2–5 min) 4 mg q 12 h, po 8 mg q 12 h (L) [Inj; T: 4, 8, 24; S: 4 mg/5 mL], but costly; see also **Table 35**.
- Spasm, pain, and vomiting: scopolamine IM, IV, SC 0.3–0.65 mg q 4–6 h prn; oral 0.4–0.8 mg q 4–8 h prn; transdermal 2.5 cm^2 patch applied behind the ear q 3 d (L) [Inj; T: 0.4; patch 1.5 mg] or hyoscyamine (*Levsin/SL*) sublingual [T: 0.125; S: 0.125 mg/mL] 0.125–0.25 tid–qid.
- Diarrhea and excessive secretions: loperamide (*Imodium A-D*) see **Table 36**; octreotide (*Sandostatin*) SC 0.15–0.3 mg q 12 h (L) [Inj], very expensive.
- Pain: see **Table 59**.
- Inflammation due to malignant obstruction: dexamethasone (*Decadron*) oral: 4 mg qid × 5–7 d.

Excessive Secretions
Nonpharmacologic: Positioning and suctioning, as needed
Pharmacologic: Glycopyrrolate 0.1–0.4 mg IV/SC q 4 h prn *or* scopolomine 0.3–0.6 mg SC prn *or* transdermal scopolomine patch q 72 h *or* atropine 0.3–0.5 mg SC, sublingual, nebulized q 4 h prn

Cough See Respiratory Diseases (p 145).

Nausea, Vomiting See Gastrointestinal Diseases (p 63).

Malnutrition, Dehydration See also Malnutrition (p 92).
Nonpharmacologic:
• Educate patient and family on effects of disease progression resulting in lack of appetite and weight loss.
• Promote interest, enjoyment in meals (eg, alcoholic beverage if desired, involve patient in meal planning, small frequent feedings, cold or semi-frozen nutritional drinks).
• Good oral care is important.
Pharmacologic:
• Corticosteroids: Dexamethasone 1–2 mg po tid; methylprednisolone 1–2 mg po bid; prednisone 5 mg po tid.
• Hormone therapy: Megestrol acetate 200–800 mg qd.

Altered Mental Status, Delirium See Delirium (p 39).

Anxiety, Depression
• Provide opportunity to discuss feelings, fears, existential concerns
• Referral to appropriate team members (spiritual, nursing)
• Medicate (see Anxiety, p 20, and Depression, p 46).

Source: Fine P. *Hospice Companion—Processes to Optimize Care During the Last Phase of Life.* 2d ed. Scottsdale, AZ: VistaCare, Inc.; 2000.

PREOPERATIVE CARE
Cardiac Risk Assessment

Figure 9. Reducing Cardiac Risk in Noncardiac Surgery

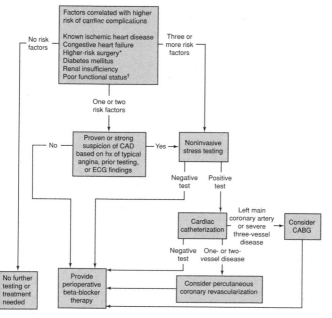

* Intraperitoneal, intrathoracic, or suprainguinal vascular procedures
† Inability to walk 4 blocks or climb 2 flights of stairs

Source: Adapted from Fleisher LA, Eagle KA. Lowering cardiac risk in noncardiac surgery. *N Engl J Med* 2001; 345:1677–1682. Copyright © 2001, Massachusetts Medical Society. All rights reserved. Adapted with permission 2003.

Pulmonary Risk Assessment
Assessing the patient for risk of pulmonary complications (respiratory failure, pneumonia, atelectasis) includes the following risk factors:
Smoking: To lower risk, patients should quit at least 8 wk before surgery.

COPD: Bronchodilators, physical therapy, antibiotics, and corticosteroids given preoperatively can reduce risk.

ASA Class: III—severe systemic disease; IV—life-threatening systemic disease; V—moribund.

Surgical Site: Upper abdominal, thoracic, > 3-h surgeries pose the greatest increased risk.

Note: Routine spirometry has not been shown to be useful in risk assessment.

Other Assessments

Anticoagulation Status: See pp 17–19.

Cognitive Status: Unrecognized dementia is a risk factor for postoperative delirium. Measure preoperative cognitive status with Mini-Cog (see p 183) or MMSE.

Nutritional Status: Poor nutritional status can impair wound healing. Measure height, weight, serum albumin.

Routine Laboratory Tests: Recommended: Hemoglobin and hematocrit, electrolytes, creatinine, BUN, ECG, CXR, albumin. Optional: CBC, platelets, ABG, PT, PTT.

Cataract Surgery: Routine laboratory testing or cardiopulmonary risk assessment is unneccessary for cataract surgery performed under local anesthesia.

Advance Directives: Establish or update.

PERIOPERATIVE MANAGEMENT

β-Blocker Use

For patients at risk for cardiac complications (see **Figure 9**), begin β-blocker agent (eg, atenolol or bisoprolol) orally 1–2 wk before surgery to achieve heart rate < 70 beats/min. Continue therapy until 2 wk after surgery, with a goal of < 80 beats/min in the postoperative period. Withhold β-blockers if heart rate is < 55 beats/min; SBP < 100; or the patient has asthma, decompensated HF, or third degree heart block.

Endocarditis Prophylaxis

Depends on cardiac condition and type of procedure (see pp 134–136).

DVT Prophylaxis (see **Table 12**)

Common Problems to Monitor

- Confusion: see p 39
- Intra- and postoperative coronary events: postoperative ECG to check
- Malnutrition: see p 92
- Pain: see p 119
- Polypharmacy: review medications daily
- Pulmonary complications: minimized by incentive spirometry, coughing, early ambulation
- Rehabilitation: encourage early mobility
- Skin breakdown: see p 157

DISCHARGE PLANNING

- Ideally, all team members should participate in discharge planning, beginning early in the hospitalization.
- Physician/general practitioner should provide discharge summary and orders, including medications.
- Site of post-discharge care should be warranted by patient's needs (see **Table 61**).
- See also Housing Alternatives, p 5.

Table 61. Sites of Post-Hospital Care		
Site	**Requirements**	**Funding**
Inpatient Rehabilitation Facility or Transitional Care Unit of a Nursing Home	Patient can tolerate 3 h of rehabilitation therapy/d requiring multiple disciplines (eg, PT, OT, speech therapy)	Medicare Part A pays 100% of charges for days 1–20, patient pays $105/d for days 21–100 with Part A covering the rest, patient pays 100% after day 100
Skilled Nursing Facility	Patient requires skilled nursing care and cannot tolerate 3 h of therapy/day	Same as above for rehabilitation services associated with hospitalization; long-term stays principally financed out-of-pocket or by Medicaid
Homebound	Physician must certify that patient is able to only occasionally leave the home at great effort	Medicare Part A pays for most non-physician professional services (eg, nursing, OT, PT); very limited coverage for attendant care (eg, cooking, cleaning)
Home/Assisted Living	Patient able to manage ADLs independently or with informal help	Medicare Part B pays for 80% of most outpatient medical services
Hospice (home or facility-based); see also p 5.	Physician must certify that patient's life expectancy < 6 mo	Medicare Part A pays for most professional services and medications related to terminal illness; physician services covered under Part B

PREVENTION

PREVENTIVE TESTS AND PROCEDURES

Table 62. Recommended Primary and Secondary Disease Prevention for Persons Aged 65 and Over

Preventive Strategy	Frequency
USPSTF* Recommendations for Primary Prevention	
Bone densitometry (women)	at least once after age 65
BP screening	yearly
Influenza immunization	yearly
Lipid disorder screening	every 5 yr, more often in CAD, diabetes mellitus, peripheral arterial disease, prior stroke
Obesity (height and weight)	yearly
Pneumonia immunization	once at age 65**
Smoking cessation	at every office visit
Tetanus immunization	every 10 yr
USPSTF* Recommendations for Secondary Prevention	
Alcohol abuse screening	unspecified but should be done periodically
Depression screening	unspecified but should be done periodically
FOBT and/or sigmoidoscopy or colonoscopy	yearly/every 3–5 yr/every 10 yr
Hearing impairment screening	yearly
Mammography, clinical breast examination***	every 1–2 yr
Pap smear†	at least every 3 yr
Visual impairment screening	yearly
Other‡ Recommendations for Primary Prevention	
Aspirin to prevent MI	daily
Diabetes mellitus screening	yearly
Omega-3 fatty acids to prevent MI, stroke	at least 2x/wk (see p 26)
Other‡ Recommendations for Secondary Prevention	
Skin examination	yearly
Breast self-examination	monthly
Cognitive impairment screening	yearly
PSA and digital rectal examination	yearly
TSH in women	yearly

* US Preventive Services Task Force. See www.ahrq.gov/clinic/uspstfix.htm
** Consider repeating pneumococcal vaccine every 6–7 yr.
*** Mammograms to age 70 are virtually universally recommended; many organizations, including the USPSTF, recommend that mammography should be continued in women over 70 who have a reasonable life expectancy.
† Pap smear testing can be stopped in most women after age 65. See p 179.
‡ Not endorsed by USPSTF for all older adults, but recommended in selected patients or by other professional organizations.

ENDOCARDITIS PROPHYLAXIS (AHA GUIDELINES)
Antibiotic Regimens Recommended (see Table 63)

Cardiac Conditions Requiring Prophylaxis
High-Risk Category: Prosthetic heart valves, previous endocarditis, surgical systemic pulmonary shunts

Moderate-Risk Category: Acquired valvular dysfunction (eg, rheumatic heart disease), hypertrophic cardiomyopathy, mitral valve prolapse with valvular regurgitation and/or thickened leaflets, most congenital heart malformations

Procedures Warranting Prophylaxis

Dental: Extractions, periodontal procedures, implants and reimplants, root canals, subgingival placement of antibiotic fibers or strips, initial placement of orthodontic bands but not brackets, intraligamentary local anesthetic injections, teeth cleaning where bleeding is expected

Respiratory Tract: Tonsillectomy and/or adenoidectomy, rigid bronchoscopy, surgery involving respiratory mucosa

GI Tract: Esophageal varices sclerotherapy, esophageal stricture dilation, endoscopic retrograde cholangiography with biliary obstruction, biliary tract surgery, surgery involving intestinal mucosa

GU Tract: Prostatic surgery, cystoscopy, urethral dilation

Cardiac Conditions Not Requiring Prophylaxis

Previous CABG surgery; mitral valve prolapse without valvular regurgitation; physiologic, functional, or innocent heart murmurs; previous rheumatic fever without valvular dysfunction; cardiac pacemakers; implanted defibrillators; isolated secundum atrial septal defect; surgical repair of atrial or ventricular septal defect

Procedures Not Warranting Prophylaxis

Dental: Restorative dentistry, local anesthetic injections, intracanal endodontic treatment, rubber dam placement, suture removal, placement of removable prosthodontic or orthodontic appliances, oral impressions, fluoride treatments, oral radiographs, orthodontic appliance adjustment

Respiratory Tract: Endotracheal intubation, flexible bronchoscopy (prophylaxis optional for high-risk patients), ear tube insertion

GI Tract: Transesophageal echocardiography, endoscopy (prophylaxis optional for high-risk patients)

GU Tract: Vaginal hysterectomy (prophylaxis optional for high-risk patients), urethral catheterization of uninfected tissue

Other: Cardiac catheterization, balloon angioplasty

Table 63. Endocarditis Prophylaxis Regimens	
Situation	**Regimen**
Dental, oral, respiratory tract, or esophageal procedures	
Standard general prophylaxis	Amoxicillin 2.0 g po 1 h before procedure
Unable to take oral medications	Ampicillin 2.0 g IM or IV $\leq$ 30 min before procedure
Allergic to penicillin	Clindamycin 600 mg or cephalexin 2.0 g or cefadroxil 2.0 g or azithromycin 500 mg or clarithromycin 500 mg po 1 h before procedure
Allergic to penicillin and unable to take oral medications	Clindamycin 600 mg or cefazolin 1.0 g IM or IV $\leq$ 30 min before procedure

(*continues*)

Table 63. Endocarditis Prophylaxis Regimens (cont.)	
Situation	Regimen
GU or GI procedures	
High-risk patients	Ampicillin 2.0 g IM or IV + 1 gentamicin 1.5 mg/kg IV or IM (not to exceed 120 mg) $\leq$ 30 min before procedure; 6 h later, ampicillin 1.0 g IM or IV or amoxicillin 1.0 g po
High-risk patients allergic to ampicillin or amoxicillin	Vancomycin 1.0 g IV over 1–2 h + gentamicin 1.5 mg/kg IV or IM (not to exceed 120 mg); complete injection or infusion $\leq$ 30 min before procedure
Moderate-risk patients	Amoxicillin 2.0 g po 1 h before procedure or ampicillin 2.0 g IM or IV $\leq$ 30 min before procedure
Moderate-risk patients allergic to ampicillin or amoxicillin	Vancomycin 1.0 g IV over 1–2 h, complete infusion $\leq$ 30 min before procedure

Note: See **Table 46** for details about antibiotics.
Source: Dajani AS, Taubert KA, Wilson W, et al. Prevention of bacterial endocarditis: Recommendations by the American Heart Association. *JAMA.* 1997;277:1794–1801. Copyright 1997, American Medical Association. Reprinted with permission.

PROPHYLAXIS FOR DENTAL PATIENTS WITH TOTAL JOINT REPLACEMENTS (TJR)

Conditions Requiring: Inflammatory arthropathies (eg, rheumatoid arthritis, systemic lupus erythematosus); disease-, drug-, or radiation-induced immunosuppression; type 1 diabetes mellitus; first 2 yr following joint replacement; previous prosthetic joint infection; malnourishment; hemophilia

Conditions Not Requiring: Patients > 2 yr post-TJR who do not have one of the above conditions; patients with pins, plates, or screws

Dental Procedures Warranting: see those listed on p 135 for endocarditis

Suggested Prophylactic Regimens: (all given 1 h before procedure)

• Not allergic to penicillin: Amoxicillin, cephalexin, or cephradine 2.0 g po
• Not allergic to penicillin and unable to take oral medications: Ampicillin 2.0 g or cefazolin 1.0 g IM or IV
• Allergic to penicillin: Clindamycin 600 mg po
• Allergic to penicillin and unable to take oral medications: Clindamycin 600 mg IV

Source: Modified from American Dental Association and American Academy of Orthopaedic Surgeons. Antibiotic prophylaxis for dental patients with total joint replacements. *JADA.* 1997;128(7):1004–1007. Copyright © 1997 American Dental Association. All rights reserved. Adapted 2003 with permission.

EXERCISE PRESCRIPTION

Before Giving an Exercise Prescription

Screen patient for:

• Musculoskeletal problems: Decreased flexibility, muscular rigidity, weakness, pain, ill-fitting shoes
• Cardiac disease: Consider stress test if patient is beginning a vigorous exercise program and is sedentary with $\geq$ 2 cardiac risk factors (male gender, hypertension, smoking, diabetes mellitus, dyslipidemia, obesity, family hx, sedentary life style).

Individualize the Prescription

Specify short- and long-term goals; include the following components:

Flexibility: Static stretching; daily, > 15 sec per muscle group

Endurance: Walking, cycling, swimming at 50%–75% of maximum HR (220 – age for men; 220 – [0.6 × age] for women); 3–4 ×/wk; goal of 20–30 min duration

Strength: Muscle resistance (weight training); 3 sets (8–15 repetitions) per muscle group 2–3 ×/wk

Balance: Tai Chi, dance, postural awareness; 1–3 ×/wk

Patient Information: See www.nia.nih.gov/exercisebook/

See also Assessment and Management of Falls, p 59.

PSYCHOTIC DISORDERS

DIAGNOSIS
Differential Diagnosis
- Bipolar affective disorder
- Delirium
- Dementia
- Drugs: eg, antiparkinsonian agents, anticholinergics, benzodiazepines or alcohol (including withdrawal), stimulants, corticosteroids, cardiac drugs (eg, digitalis), opioid analgesics
- Late-life delusional (paranoid) disorder
- Major depression
- Physical disorders: hypo- or hyperglycemia, hypo- or hyperthyroidism, sodium or potassium imbalance, Cushing's syndrome, Parkinson's disease, B_{12} deficiency, sleep deprivation, AIDS
- Pain, untreated
- Schizophrenia
- Structural brain lesions: tumor or stroke
- Seizure disorder: eg, temporal lobe

Risk Factors for Psychotic Symptoms in Elderly Persons
Chronic bed rest, cognitive impairment, female gender, sensory impairment, social isolation

MANAGEMENT
- Alleviate underlying physical causes.
- Address identifiable psychosocial triggers.
- If psychotic symptoms are severe, frightening, or may affect safety, use antipsychotic.
- Olanzapine, quetiapine, risperidone are first choice because of fewer side effects (TD extremely high in elderly patients taking typical antipsychotics).

Table 64. Representative Antipsychotic Medications			
Class, Agent	Dosage*	Formulations	Comments (Metabolism)
Atypical Antipsychotics			
Aripiprazole (*Abilify*)	10–15 (1) initially; max 30/d	T: 10, 15, 20, 30	Very limited geriatrics experience; potential for somnolence; wait 2 wk between dose changes (CYP2D6, 3A4) (L)
Clozapine (*Clozaril*)	25–150 (1)	T: 25, 100	May be useful for parkinsonism and TD; sedation, orthostasis, anticholinergic, agranulocytosis, weight gain (L)
✓ Olanzapine (*Zyprexa*)	2.5–10 (1)	T: 2.5, 5, 7.5, 10, 15, 20; disintegrating tab: 5, 10, 15, 20	Sedation, anticholinergic effects at high doses, weight gain, hyperglycemia, risk of diabetes; dose-related EPS (L)

Table 64. Representative Antipsychotic Medications (cont.)			
Class, Agent	Dosage*	Formulations	Comments (Metabolism)
✓ Quetiapine (*Seroquel*)	25–800 (1–2)	T: 25, 100, 200, 300	Sedation, orthostasis, no dose-related EPS (L, K)
✓ Risperidone (*Risperdal*)	0.5–1 (1–2)	T: 0.25, 0.5, 1, 2, 3, 4 scored; S: 1 mg/mL	Orthostasis, dose-related EPS, caution in patients at risk of stroke; do not exceed 6 mg (L, K)
Ziprasidone (*Geodon*)	20–80 (1–2)	C: 20, 40, 60, 80	May increase QT$_c$; very limited geriatric data (L)
Low Potency			
Thioridazine (eg, *Mellaril*)	25–200 (1–3)	T: 10, 15, 25, 50, 100, 150, 200; S: 30 mg/mL	Anticholinergic, orthostasis, QT$_c$ prolongation, sedation, TD; for acute use only (L, K)
Intermediate Potency			
Loxapine (*Loxitane*)	2.5–20 (1–3)	C: 5, 10, 25, 50; S: 25 mg/mL	Anticholinergic, orthostasis, sedation, TD; for acute use only (L, K)
High Potency			
Haloperidol (*Haldol*)	0.5–2 (1–3); depot 100–200 mg IM q 4 wk	T: 0.5, 1, 2, 5, 10, 20; S: conc 2 mg/mL; Inj	EPS, TD; for acute use only (L, K)

*Total mg/d (frequency/d).
Note: ✓ = preferred for treating older persons.

Table 65. Management of Side Effects of Antipsychotic Medications		
Side Effect	Treatment	Comment
Drug-induced parkinsonism	Lower dose or switch to atypical antipsychotic	Often dose related
Akathisia (motor restlessness)	Switch to atypical antipsychotic, β-blocker (eg, propranolol [*Inderal*] 20–40 mg/d) or low-dose benzodiazepine (eg, lorazepam 0.5 mg bid)	Also seen with atypical antipsychotics; more likely with traditional agents
Hypotension	Slow titration; reduce dose; change drug class	More common with low-potency agents
Sedation	Reduce dose; give at bedtime; change drug class	More common with low-potency agents
TD	Stop drug (if possible); change to atypical antipsychotic	Increased risk in elderly; may be irreversible

Note: Periodic (q 4 mo) reevaluation of antipsychotic dose and ongoing need is important (see OBRA Regulations, p 197). Older persons are particularly sensitive to side effects of antipsychotic drugs. They are also at higher risk of developing TD. Periodic use of a side-effect scale such as the AIMS (see p 189) is highly recommended.

ACUTE RENAL FAILURE
Definition
An acute deterioration in renal function defined by decreased urine output or increased values of renal function tests, or both

Precipitating and Aggravating Factors
- Acute tubular necrosis due to hypoperfusion or nephrotoxins
- Medications (eg, aminoglycosides, radiocontrast materials, NSAIDs, ACE inhibitors)
- Multiple myeloma
- Obstruction (eg, BPH)
- Vascular disease (thromboembolic, atheroembolic)
- Volume depletion or redistribution of extracellular fluid (eg, cirrhosis, burns)

Evaluation
- Review medication list
- Catheterize bladder, determine postvoid residual
- Perform UA
- Perform renal ultrasonography
- Determine fractional excretion of sodium (FENa):

$$FENa = \frac{urine\ Na/plasma\ Na \times 100\%}{urine\ creatinine/plasma\ creatinine}$$

(*FENa < 1% indicates prerenal cause; FENa > 3% indicates acute tubular necrosis; FENa 1%–3% is nondiagnostic. Note that some older persons who have prerenal cause may have FENa ≥ 1% because of age-related changes in sodium excretion.*)

Treatment
- D/C medications that are possible precipitants; avoid contrast dyes.
- If prerenal pattern, treat HF if present (see p 26). Otherwise, volume repletion. Begin with fluid challenge 500–1000 cc over 30–60 min. If no response, give furosemide 100–400 mg IV.
- If obstructed, leave bladder catheter in place while evaluation and specific treatment are being implemented.
- If acute tubular necrosis, monitor weights daily, record intake and output, and monitor electrolytes frequently. Fluid replacement should be equal to urinary output plus other drainage plus 500 cc/d for insensible losses.
- Dialysis is indicated when severe hyperkalemia, acidosis, or volume overload cannot be managed with other therapies or when uremic symptoms (eg, pericarditis, coagulopathy, or encephalopathy) are present.

VOLUME DEPLETION (DEHYDRATION)
Definition
Losses of sodium and water that may be isotonic (eg, loss of blood) or hypotonic (eg, nasogastric suctioning)

Precipitating Factors

- Blood loss
- Diuretics
- GI losses
- Renal or adrenal disease (eg, renal sodium wasting)
- Sequestration of fluid (eg, ileus, burns, peritonitis)
- Age-related changes (impaired thirst, sodium wasting due to hyporeninemic hypoaldosteronism, and free water wasting due to renal insensitivity to antidiuretic hormone)

Evaluation

Clinical symptoms:

- Anorexia
- Nausea and vomiting
- Orthostatic lightheadedness
- Delirium
- Weakness

Clinical signs:

- Dry tongue and axillae oliguria
- Orthostatic hypotension
- Elevated heart rate
- Weight loss

Laboratory Tests

- Serum electrolytes
- Urine sodium (usually < 10 mEq/L) and FENa (usually < 1% but may be higher because of age-related sodium wasting)
- Serum BUN and creatinine (BUN/creatinine ratio often > 20)

Management

- Daily weight; monitor fluid losses and serum electrolytes, BUN, creatinine
- If mild, oral rehydration of 2–4 L of water/d and 4–8 g Na diet; if poor oral intake, give IV D5W1/2 NS with potassium as needed
- If hemodynamically unstable, give IV 0.9% saline 500 cc bolus and 200 cc/h until systolic BP ≥ 100 and no longer orthostatic. Then switch to D5W1/2 NS. Monitor closely in patients with a hx of HF.

HYPERNATREMIA

Causes

- Pure water loss:
  - insensible losses due to sweating and respiration
  - central (eg, post-traumatic, CNS tumors, meningitis) diabetes insipidus or nephrogenic (eg, hypercalcemia, lithium) diabetes insipidus
- Hypotonic sodium loss:
  - renal causes: osmotic diuresis (eg, due to hyperglycemia); postobstructive diuresis; polyuric phase of acute tubular necrosis
  - GI causes: vomiting and diarrhea, nasogastric drainage, osmotic cathartic agents (eg, lactulose)
- Hypertonic sodium gain (eg, treatment with hypertonic saline)
- Impaired thirst (eg, delirious or intubated) or access to water (eg, functionally dependent) may sustain hypernatremia

Evaluation
- Measure intake and output.
- Obtain urine osmolality:
  - \> 800 mOsm/kg suggests extrarenal (if urine Na < 25 mEq/L) or remote renal water loss or administration of hypertonic Na^+ salt solutions (if urine Na > 100 mEq/L).
  - < 250 mOsm/kg and polyuria suggest diabetes insipidus.

Treatment
- Treat underlying causes.
- Correct slowly over at least 48–72 h using oral (can use pure water), nasogastric (can use pure water), or IV (D5W, 1/2 or 1/4 NS) fluids; correct at rate of no more than 1 mmol/L/h if acute (eg, developing over hours) and at no more than 10 mmol/L/d if of longer duration.
- Correct with normal saline only in cases of severe volume depletion with hemodynamic compromise; once stable, switch to hypotonic solution.
- When repleting, use the following formula to estimate the effect of 1 L of any infusate on serum Na:

$$\text{Change in serum Na} = \frac{\text{infusate Na} - \text{serum Na}}{\text{total body water} + 1}$$

- Infusate Na (mmol/L): D5W = 0; 1/4 NS = 34; 1/2 NS = 77; NS = 154.
- Calculate total body water as a fraction of body weight (0.5 kg in older men and 0.45 kg in older women).
- Divide treatment goal (usually 10 mmol/L/d) by change in serum Na/L (from formula) to determine amount of solution to be given over 24 h.
- Compensate for any ongoing obligatory fluid losses, which are usually 1.0–1.5 L/d.
- Divide amount of solution for repletion plus amount for obligatory fluid losses by 24 to determine rate per h.

HYPONATREMIA
Causes
- With increased plasma osmolality: Hyperglycemia (1.6 mEq/L decrement for each 100 mg/dL increase in plasma glucose)
- With normal plasma osmolality (pseudohyponatremia): Severe hyperlipidemia, hyperproteinemia (eg, multiple myeloma)
- With decreased plasma osmolality:
  - With extracellular fluid (ECF) excess: Renal failure, heart failure, hepatic cirrhosis, nephrotic syndrome
  - With decreased ECF volume: Renal losses from salt-losing nephropathies, diuretics, osmotic diuresis, extrarenal loss due to vomiting, diarrhea, skin losses, and third-spacing (usually urine Na < 20 mEq/L, FENa < 1%, and uric acid > 4 mg/dL)
  - With normal ECF volume: Primary polydipsia (urine osmolarity < 100 mOsm/kg), hypothyroidism, adrenal insufficiency, SIADH (urine Na > 40 mEq/L and uric acid < 4 mg/dL)

Management

Only if symptomatic (eg, altered mental status, seizures) or severe acute hyponatremia (eg, < 120 mEq/L):

- Goal is 0.5 mEq/L/h rise in Na (more rapid correction can result in central pontine myelinolysis); time (in hours) to correct = $(140 - Na)/0.5$ mEq/L/h.
- Calculate free water excess (liters) = $(0.5 \times$ current body weight in kg$) \times (1 - [Na/140])$.
- Target rate of free water removal (L/h) = free water excess/time to correct.
- Replace urine output with 3% saline or isotonic saline.
- Monitor Na closely and taper treatment when > 120 or symptoms resolve.

SIADH
Definition

Hypotonic hyponatremia (< 280 mOsm/kg) with:
- Less than maximally dilute urine (usually > 100 mOsm/kg)
- Elevated urine sodium (usually > 40 mEq/L)
- Normal volume status
- Normal renal, adrenal, and thyroid function

Precipitating Factors, Causes

- Drugs (eg, SSRIs, venlafaxine, chlorpropamide, carbamazepine, NSAIDs, barbiturates)
- Neuropsychiatric factors (eg, neoplasm, subarachnoid hemorrhage, psychosis, meningitis)
- Postoperative state, especially if pain or nausea
- Pulmonary disease (eg, pneumonia, tuberculosis, acute asthma)
- Tumors (eg, lung, pancreas, thymus)

Evaluation

- BUN, creatinine, serum cortisol, TSH
- CXR
- Review of medications
- Neurologic tests as indicated
- Urine sodium and osmolality

Management

Acute Treatment: See hyponatremia management (above)
Chronic Treatment:
- D/C offending drug or treat precipitating illness.
- Restrict water to 1000–1500 mL/d.
- Liberalize salt intake.
- Demeclocycline (*Declomycin*) 150–300 mg bid [T: 150, 300] (may be nephrotoxic in patients with liver disease).

BENIGN PROSTATIC HYPERPLASIA
Evaluation

Detailed medical hx focusing on the urinary tract physical examination, including a digital rectal examination and a focused neurologic examination; UA; measurement of serum creatinine. Measurement of PSA is optional.

Management

Mild Symptoms: (eg, AUA score $\leq$ 7; see p 195) watchful waiting

Moderate to Severe Symptoms: (eg, AUA score $\geq$ 8; see p 195) medical or surgical treatment

Medical Treatment: Combining drugs from different classes may be more effective than single-agent therapy

- α_1-Blockers:
  - Terazosin (*Hytrin*) advance as tolerated—days 1–3, 1 mg/d hs; days 4–7, 2 mg; days 8–14, 5 mg; day 15 and beyond, 10 mg [T: 1, 2, 5, 10]
  - Doxazosin (*Cardura*) start 0.5 mg with max of 16 mg/d [T: 1, 2, 4, 8]
  - Prazosin (*Minipress*) start 1 mg/d (first dose hs) or bid with max 20 mg/d [T: 1, 2, 5]
  - Tamsulosin (*Flomax*) 0.4 mg half-hour after the same meal each day and increase to 0.8 mg if no response in 2–4 wk [T: 0.4]
- 5-α Reductase inhibitors:
  - Finasteride (*Proscar*) 5 mg/d [T: 5]
  - Dutasteride (*Avodart*) 0.5 mg/d [C: 0.5]

Surgical Management: Indicated if recurrent UTI, recurrent or persistent gross hematuria, bladder stones, or renal insufficiency are clearly secondary to BPH or as indicated by symptoms, patient preference, or failure of medical treatment. Options are:

- Transurethral resection of the prostate (TURP).
- Transurethral incision of the prostate (TUIP), which is limited to prostates whose estimated resected tissue weight (if done by TURP) would be 30 g or less.
- Open prostatectomy for large glands.

Source: McConnell JD, Barry MJ, Bruskewitz RC, et al. *Benign Prostatic Hyperplasia: Diagnosis and Treatment.* Clinical Practice Guideline No. 8. Rockville, MD: Agency for Health Care Policy and Research, Public Health Service, US Dept. of Health and Human Services, February 1994. AHCPR Publication No. 94-0582.

PROSTATE CANCER(see p 77)

ALLERGIC RHINITIS

Definition

- The most common atopic disorder.
- Symptoms include rhinorrhea; sneezing; and irritated eyes, nose, and mucous membranes.
- May be seasonal, but in older people is more often perennial.
- Postnasal drip, mainly from chronic rhinitis, is the most common cause of chronic cough.

Therapy

Nonpharmacologic: Avoid allergens, eliminate pets and their dander, dehumidify to reduce molds; reduce outdoor exposures during pollen season; reduce house dust mites by encasing pillows and mattresses. Arachnocides reduce mites.

Pharmacologic: Target therapy to symptoms and on whether symptoms are seasonal or perennial; see **Table 66** and **Table 67**.

Table 66. Choosing Therapy for Allergic Nasal Symptoms				
Agent or Class	**Rhinitis**	**Sneezing**	**Pruritus**	**Congestion**
Glucocorticoids*	+	+	+	+
Ipratropium*	+			
Antihistamines**†	+	+	+	
Pseudoephedrine‡				+
Cromolyn†	+	+	+	+

* Effective in seasonal, perennial, and vasomotor rhinitis.
** Better in seasonal than in perennial rhinitis.
† Start before allergy season.
‡ Topical therapy rapid in onset but results in rebound if used for more than a few days; facilitates use of nasal steroids and sleep during severe attacks.

Table 67. Drug Therapy for Allergic Rhinitis				
Type, Drug	**Geriatric Dosage**	**Formulations**	**Geriatric Half-Life**	**Side Effects**
H₁-Receptor Antagonists or Antihistamines				
√Azelastine (*Astelin*)	2 spr bid**	topical spr 0.1%, 100 spr	22–25 h	Bitter taste, nasal burning, sneezing
√Cetirizine (*Zyrtec*)	5 mg/d (max)	T: 5, 10; syr 5 mg/ 5 mL	Prolonged	
√Desloratadine (*Clarinex*)	5 mg	T: 5	27 h	
Fexofenadine (√*Allegra*, *Allegra-D**)	60 mg po bid; once a day if CrCl < 40; D not recommended	T: 30, 60, 180; C: 60	14 h	

(continues)

Table 67. Drug Therapy for Allergic Rhinitis (cont.)				
Type, Drug	Geriatric Dosage	Formulations	Geriatric Half-Life	Side Effects
Loratadine (√Claritin, Claritin-D,* generic, OTC)	5–10 mg qd; D not recommended	T: 10; rapid-disintegrating tab 10 mg; syr 1 mg/mL	Metabolites > 12 d; wide variation	
Chlorpheniramine (eg, Chlor-Trimeton)	8–12 mg bid	T: 4, 8, 12; ChT: 2; CR: 8, 12; S: 2 mg/ 5 mL	20 h, longer with renal dysfunction	Sedation, dry mouth, confusion, urinary retention; dries lung secretions
Diphenhydramine (eg, Benadryl)	25–50 mg bid	T: 25, 50; S: elixir 12.5 mg/mL	13.5 h	Same as chlorpheniramine
Hydroxyzine (eg, Atarax)	25–30 mg bid	T: 10, 25, 50	30 h	Same as chlorpheniramine
Decongestants				
Pseudoephedrine (eg, Sudafed, combinations)	60 mg po q 4–6 h	T: 30, 60; SR: 120; S: elixir 30 mg/5 mL	2–16 h; varies with urine pH	Arrhythmia, insomnia, anxiety, restlessness, elevated BP
Nasal Steroids				Class side effects:
Beclomethasone (eg, Beconase, Vancenase)	1 spr bid–qid**	topical spr 16 g (80 spr)	Rapid absorption, hepatic metabolism	nasal burning, sneezing, bleeding; septal perforation (rare); fungal overgrowth (rare); no significant systemic effects
Budesonide (eg, Rhinocort)	2 spr bid or 4 qd**	7 g (200 spr)		
Dexamethasone (eg, Dexacort)	2 spr bid or tid**	25 mL (200 spr)		
Flunisolide (eg, Nasalide, Nasarel)	2–4 spr bid or tid**	25 mL (200 spr)		
Fluticasone (eg, Flonase)	2 spr qd**	16 g (120 spr)		
Mometasone (Nasonex)	2 spr qd**	17 g (120 spr)		
Triamcinolone (eg, Nasacort)	2–4 spr qd**	10 g (100 spr)		
Other				
Cromolyn (NasalCrom)	1 spr tid–qid;** begin 1–2 wk before exposure to allergen	2%, 4%		Nasal irritation, headache, itching of throat

Table 67. Drug Therapy for Allergic Rhinitis (cont.)				
Type, Drug	Geriatric Dosage	Formulations	Geriatric Half-Life	Side Effects
Ipratropium (*Atrovent NS*)	2 spr bid–qid**	0.03, 0.06%† sol	1.6 h	Epistaxis, nasal irritation, URI, sore throat, nausea. Caution: Do not spray in eyes.
Montelukast (*Singulair*)	10 mg po qd	T: 10 mg; gran 4 mg/packet		Less effective than nasal steroids

Note: √ = preferred for treating older persons.
* *Allegra-D, Claritin-D* are not recommended; both also contain pseudoephedrine. Contraindicated in narrow angle glaucoma, urinary retention, MAOI use within 14 d, severe hypertension, or CAD. May cause headache, nausea, insomnia.
** Spr per nares.
† Use 0.06% for treatment of viral upper respiratory infection.

CHRONIC OBSTRUCTIVE PULMONARY DISEASE
Definition
A spectrum of chronic respiratory diseases characterized by:
- Airflow limitation
- Cough
- Dyspnea
- Frequent pulmonary infection
- Impaired gas exchange
- Sputum production

Therapy
Smoking Cessation: Essential at any age. See p 15.
Rehabilitation: Patients at all stages benefit from exercise training, ie, increased exercise tolerance results in decreased dyspnea and fatigue.
Long-Term Oxygen Therapy: For indications, see **Table 72**.
MDIs: Should be used with an aerochamber; educate patients on use. Use a separate aerochamber for inhaled steroids; wash aerochamber weekly; aerochamber requires separate prescription.
Stepped Approach: Add steps when symptoms inadequately controlled; D/C agent if no improvement. See **Table 68** and **Table 71**.

Table 68. COPD Therapy	
Stage	Treatment
Mild COPD FEV $\geq$ 80%	Short-acting β_2-agonist when needed
Moderate COPD	
50% $\leq$ FEV < 80%	Regular treatment with one or more bronchodilators* Rehabilitation Inhaled steroids if significant symptoms and lung function response
30% $\leq$ FEV < 50%	Regular treatment with one or more bronchodilators* Rehabilitation Inhaled steroids if significant symptoms and lung function response or if repeated exacerbations

(*continues*)

Table 68. COPD Therapy (cont.)	
Stage	**Treatment**
Severe COPD	Regular treatment with one or more bronchodilators*
FEV < 30% or respiratory or right HF	Inhaled steroids if significant symptoms and lung function response or if repeated exacerbations
	Treatment of complications
	Long-term O_2 therapy if respiratory failure
COPD exacerbation	Increase dose and/or frequency of bronchodilators*
(increased breathlessness, wheezing, cough, sputum)	Consider IV methylxanthine
	Add steroid (eg, methylprednisolone 30–40 mg po qd 10–14 d)
	Add antibiotics if ↑ sputum with ↑ purulence (cover *Streptococcus pneumoniae, Haemophilus influenzae, Moraxella catarrhalis*)
	Check x-ray, ECG, ABG; titrate O_2 to 90% sat and recheck ABG
	If ≥ 2: severe dyspnea, respiratory rate ≥ 25, pCO_2 45–60, then noninvasive positive pressure ventilation reduces risk of ventilator use and mortality and length of hospital stay

* β_2-agonists, ipratropium, methylxanthines

Source: Adapted from Global Strategy for the Diagnosis, Management, and Prevention of Chronic Obstructive Pulmonary Disease, Global Initiative for Chronic Obstructive Lung Disease (GOLD). NHLBI/WHO Workshop Report, Executive Summary. National Institutes of Health, National Heart, Lung and Blood Institute. March 2001. NIH Publication No. 2701A (for full report, see www.goldcopd.com).

ASTHMA
Definition
Chronic inflammatory disorder of the airways; may be triggered by:
- Air pollution
- Allergens
- Chemicals
- Emotional distress
- Exercise
- Tobacco smoke
- Viruses

Characteristics
Can present at any age, but in old age: **cough** is a common presentation, it is less variable and episodic, presents more fixed obstruction, is more difficult to classify. Symptoms:
- Chest tightness
- Cough
- Reversible and variable PEF
- Shortness of breath
- Wheezing

Symptoms may be confused with HF, COPD; PEF may not be reliable.

Therapy
Nonpharmacologic: Avoid triggers; educate patients on disease management, use of MDIs (document severity and response to therapy).
Pharmacologic: Stepped approach:
- Based on severity of symptoms.
- When symptoms controlled for 3 months, try stepwise reduction.
- If control not achieved, step up, but first review medication technique, adherence, and avoidance of triggers. (See **Table 70**, **Table 71**.)

MDIs should be used with an aerochamber, and patients should be educated on their use. Use separate aerochamber for steroids; wash aerochamber weekly; aerochamber requires separate prescription.

Table 69. Classification of Asthma Severity				
	Symptoms During Day	Symptoms at Night	PEF or FEVI	PEF Variability
Intermittent	< 1/wk; asymptomatic between attacks	< 2/mo	$\geq$ 80%	< 20%
Mild, persistent	> 2/wk; attacks may affect activity	> 2/mo	$\geq$ 80%	20–30%
Moderate, persistent	Daily, attacks affect activity	> 1/wk	60–80%	> 30%
Severe, persistent	Continual; limited physical activity	Frequent	$\leq$ 60%	> 30%

Source: Adapted from Global Initiative for Asthma, *Global Strategy for Asthma Prevention and Management*. Bethesda, MD: National Heart, Lung, and Blood Institute, April 2002. NIH Publication No. 02-3654. www.ginasthma.com

Table 70. Asthma Therapy for Adults			
	Daily Medications	Other Options	Geriatric Notes
Step 1 Intermittent	None	Inhaled β_2-agonist prn	
Step 2 Mild, persistent	Low-dose inhaled steroid	SR-theophylline or cromone or leukotriene inhibitor	Many drug interactions with theophylline; leukotrienes have not been studied in older patients
Step 3 Moderate, persistent	Low- to medium-dose inhaled steroid plus long-acting inhaled β_2-agonist	Medium-dose inhaled steroid plus SR-theophylline, or medium-dose inhaled steroid plus either oral β_2-agonist or leukotriene inhibitor, or high-dose inhaled steroid	Oral β_2-agonists cause tremors, tachycardia, angina; many older patients have fixed obstruction, and ipratropium is helpful and well tolerated
Step 4 Severe, persistent	High-dose inhaled steroid plus long-acting inhaled β_2-agonist plus one or more of SR-theophylline, leukotriene inhibitor, oral long-acting β_2-agonist, oral steroid		

Sources: Adapted from National Asthma Education and Prevention Program, *NAEPP Working Group Report: Considerations for Diagnosing and Managing Asthma in the Elderly*. Bethesda, MD: National Heart, Lung, and Blood Institute; Feb. 1996. NIH Publication No. 96-3662 and Global Initiative for Asthma, *Global Strategy for Asthma Prevention and Management*. Bethesda, MD: National Heart, Lung, and Blood Institute, April 2002. NIH Publication No. 02-3654. www.ginasthma.com

Table 71. Asthma and COPD Medications		
Drug	Dosage	Side Effects (Metabolism, Excretion)
Anticholinergics		
√ Ipratropium (*Atrovent*)	2–6 puffs qid or 0.5 mg by nebulizer qid	Dry mouth, bitter taste (Lung; poorly absorbed)
Short-acting β₂-Agonists*		Class side effects include tremor, nervousness, headache, palpitations, tachycardia, cough, hypokalemia. Caution: use half-doses in persons with known or suspected coronary disease (L)
√ Albuterol (*Proventil, Ventolin*)	2–6 puffs q 4–6 h or 2.5 mg by nebulizer qid; 1.5–3.5 mg bid–qid by nebulizer; ER tablets 4–8 mg po q 12 h	
Albuterol (*Ventolin Rotacaps*)	1–2 caps q 4–6 h; dry powder inhaler 200 μg/inhalation	
√ Bitolterol (*Tornalate*)	1–3 puffs q 4–6 h	
Isoetharine (eg, *Bronkometer, Bronkosol*)	0.25–0.5 mL of 1% sol; 2 mL NS by nebulizer q 1–4 h; inhaler 1–2 puffs q 4 h	Use limited by short duration of action; not widely used for this reason
Levalbuterol (*Xopenex*)	0.63 mg q 6–8 h	Expensive; no advantage over racemic albuterol
Pirbuterol (*Maxair*)	2–3 puffs q 4–6 h	Mechanism may be difficult for older patients to trigger
Long-acting β-Agonists		Class side effects include tremor, nervousness, headache, palpitations, tachycardia, cough, hypokalemia; caution: use half-doses in persons with known or suspected coronary disease; not for acute exacerbation (L)
Salmeterol (*Serevent Diskus*)	1 cap bid; dry powdered inhaler 50 μg/inhalation	
√ Formoterol (*Foradil*)	1 puff q 12 h	Onset of action 1–3 min
Corticosteroids: Inhaled		Class side effects include nausea, vomiting, diarrhea, abdominal pain; oropharyngeal thrush; dosages > 1.0 mg/d may cause adrenal suppression, reduce calcium absorption and bone density, and cause bruising (L)
√ Beclomethasone (*Beclovent, Vanceril*)	2–4 puffs bid–qid [42, 84 μg/puff, max 840 mg/d]	
√ Budesonide (eg, *Pulmicort*)	1–2 puffs bid–qid [100, 200, 400 μg/puff]	
√ Dexamethasone (eg, *Dexacort*)	3 puffs tid–qid [100 μg/puff]	
√ Flunisolide (eg, *AeroBid*)	2–4 puffs bid [250 μg/puff]	
√ Fluticasone (eg, *Flovent*)	1 puff bid [44, 110, 220 μg/puff]	
√ Triamcinolone (eg, *Azmacort*)	2 puffs tid–qid or 4 puffs bid [100 μg/puff]	
Corticosteroids: Oral		
Prednisone (eg, *Deltasone, Orasone*)	20 mg po bid [T: 1, 2.5, 5, 10, 20, 50; elixir 5 mg/5 mL]	Leukocytosis, thrombocytosis, sodium retention, euphoria, depression, hallucination, cognitive dysfunction; other effects with long-term use (L)

Table 71. Asthma and COPD Medications (cont.)		
Drug	Dosage	Side Effects (Metabolism, Excretion)
Methylxanthines		
Long-acting Theophyllines (eg, *Quibron-T/SR*)	300–400 mg/d [T: 300 bisect, trisect tabs]	Class side effects include atrial arrhythmias, seizures, increased gastric acid secretion, ulcer, reflux, diuresis; clearance ↓ by 30% after 65 yr; initial dose ≤ 400 mg/d, titrate using blood levels (L)
(eg, *Theo-Dur, Slo-Bid*)	100–200 mg po bid [T: 100, 200, 300, 450]	
(eg, *Uniphyl, Theo-24*)	400 mg po qd [T: 100, 200, 300, 400]	
Leukotriene Modifiers		
Montelukast (*Singulair*)	10 mg po in AM [T: 10; ChT: 4, 5]	Unknown, minimal data in elderly patients; leukotriene-receptor antagonist (L)
Zafirlukast (*Accolate*)	20 mg po bid 1 h before or 2 h after meals [T: 10, 20]	Headache, somnolence, dizziness, nausea, diarrhea, abdominal pain, fever; monitor LFTs; monitor coumarin anticoagulants; leukotriene-receptor antagonist (L, reduced by 50% > 65 yr)
Zileuton (*Zyflo*)	600 mg po qid [T: 600]	Dizziness, insomnia, nausea, abdominal pain, abnormal LFTs, myalgia; monitor coumarin anticoagulants; other drug interactions; inhibits synthesis of leukotrienes (L)
Other Medications		
√ Albuterol-Ipratropium (*Combivent*)	0.09/0.018 mg/puff, 2–3 puffs qid; 3 mg/ 0.5 mg by nebulizer qid	Same as individual agents (L, K)
Cromolyn sodium (eg, *Intal*)	2–4 puffs or 20-mg caps qid	Because of propellant, use MDI with caution in coronary disease or arrhythmia (L, K)
Nedocromil (*Tilade*)	2 puffs qid	Bitter taste, headache, dizziness, sore throat, cough, chest tightness (K, F)
Salmeterol-Fluticasone combination (*Advair Diskus*)	1 puff bid (50 μg/100, 250, or 500 μg/ inhalation)	

Note: √ = preferred for treating older persons.

* Older nonselective β_2-agonists such as isoproterenol, metoproterenol, epinephrine are not recommended and are more toxic.

Table 72. Indications for Long-Term Oxygen Therapy*		
Pao$_2$ Level	Sao$_2$ Level	Other
≤ 55 mm Hg	≤ 88%	> 15 hr/d for benefit†
55–59 mm Hg	≥ 89%	Signs of tissue hypoxia (ie, cor pulmonale by ECG, HF, hematocrit > 55%)
≥ 60 mm Hg	≥ 90%	Desaturation with exercise Desaturation with sleep apnea not corrected by CPAP

* Titrate O$_2$ saturation to approximately 90%.
† Improves survival, hemodynamics, polycythemia, exercise capacity, lung mechanics, and cognition.
Source: Adapted from Global Strategy for the Diagnosis, Management, and Prevention of Chronic Obstructive Pulmonary Disease, Global Initiative for Chronic Obstructive Lung Disease (GOLD). NHLBI/WHO Workshop Report, Executive Summary. National Institutes of Health, National Heart, Lung and Blood Institute. March 2001. NIH Publication No. 2701A (for full report, see www.goldcopd.com).

COUGH
- Symptom of acute and chronic respiratory and cardiac illnesses.
- Chronic rhinitis is most common cause in older people (see **Table 67**).

Management
- Identify cause, then treat underlying problem.
- Do not suppress cough in stable COPD.
- For symptomatic relief, see **Table 73**.
- Evaluate for side effects from other medications, eg, ACE inhibitors

Table 73. Antitussives and Expectorants			
Drug	Dosage	Formulations	Comments (Metabolism)
Benzonatate* (*Tessalon Perles*)	100 mg po tid (max: 600 mg/d)	C: 100, 200	Side effects: CNS stimulation or depression, headache, dizziness, hallucination, constipation (L)
Dextromethorphan** (eg, *Robitussin DM*)	10–30 mL po q 4–8 h	C: 30; S: 10 mg/ 5 mL	Side effects: mild drowsiness, fatigue; interacts with fluoxetine, paroxetine; combination may cause serotonin syndrome (L)
Guaifenesin** (eg, *Robitussin*)	5–20 mL po q 4 h	S: 100 mg/5 mL	Side effects: none at low doses; high doses cause nausea, vomiting, diarrhea, drowsiness, abdominal pain (L)
Histussin HC**	10 mL q 4 h up to 40 mL/d	S: hydrocodone 2.5 mg + phenylephrine 5 mg + chlor- pheniramine 2 mg/mL	Side effects: sedation, constipation, nervousness, tachycardia, hypertension, urinary retention (L)
Hydrocodone** (*Hycodan*)	5 mL po q 4–6 h	S: 5 mg/5 mL	Side effects include sedation, constipation, confusion (L)

Note: * = antitussive and expectorant; ** = antitussive.

PULMONARY EMBOLISM

Symptoms

Classic triad—dyspnea, chest pain, hemoptysis—occurs in ≤ 20% of cases. Consider PE with any of the following:

- Chest pain
- Hemoptysis
- Hypotension
- Hypoxia
- Shortness of breath
- Syncope
- Tachycardia

Diagnosis

Figure 10. Evaluation of Suspected Pulmonary Emboli

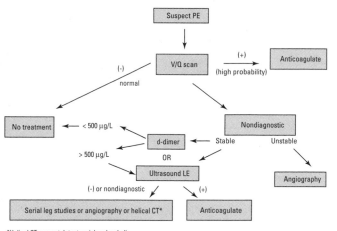

*Helical CT may not detect peripheral emboli.

Pharmacologic Therapy

- Standard therapy for PE remains IV heparin followed by warfarin.
  - Heparin: mix infusion 100 units/mL in D5W; cleared through the reticuloendothelial system, half-life of anticoagulation effect 1.5 h
  - Warfarin (see p 17 and **Table 10**)
- Low-molecular-weight heparins (LMWH) appear safe and effective for both DVT and PE. (see **Table 12**)
- Acute massive PE (filling defects in 2 or more lobar arteries, or the equivalent, by angiogram) associated with hypotension or severe hypoxia or high pulmonary pressures on ECG should usually be treated with thrombolytic therapy within 48 h of onset. (see **Table 12**)

IMPOTENCE (ERECTILE DYSFUNCTION)
Definition
Inability to achieve erection sufficient for intercourse. Prevalence nearly 70% by age 70.

Causes
Often multifactorial; > 50% of cases arterial, venous, or mixed vascular cause. Also:
- Diabetes mellitus
- Drug side effects
- Hyperprolactinemia
- Hypogonadism
- Neurologic: eg, disorders of the CNS, spinal cord, or PNS; autonomic neuropathy; temporal lobe epilepsy
- Psychologic: eg, depression, anxiety, bereavement
- Thyroid or adrenal disorders

Decreased bioavailable testosterone is more associated with decreased libido than with erectile dysfunction.

Evaluation
History: Type and duration of problem; relation to surgery, trauma, medication. Problems with orgasm, libido, or penile detumescence are not erectile dysfunction.
Physical Findings:
- Neuropathy: orthostatic hypotension, impaired response to Valsalva's maneuver, absent bulbocavernosus or cremasteric reflexes
- Peyronie's disease: penile bands, plaques
- Hypogonadism: diminished male pattern hair, gynecomastia, small (< 20–25 mm long) testes
Assessment:
- Reduced penile-to-brachial pressure index suggests vascular disease.
- Cavernosometry diagnoses venous leak syndrome; reserved for surgical candidates.
- Test dose of prostaglandin E or papaverine can exclude vascular disease or confirm venous leak syndrome.
- For libido problems check total and bioavailable testosterone, luteinizing hormone, TSH, and prolactin. Most late life hypogonadism is hypothalamic failure. Sex hormone binding globulin goes up; bioavailable testosterone is the most sensitive test.

Therapy

Table 74. Management of Male Sexual Dysfunction		
Cause	Therapy	Comments
Hypogonadism, poor libido	Testosterone: scrotal transdermal (*Testoderm*) [4, 5, 6] 4–6 mg qd; *or* skin transdermal (*Androderm*) [2.5, 5] 5 mg/d; *or* testosterone cypionate or enanthate 200 mg IM q 2–4 wk	When given IM, can cause polycythemia, fluid retention, gynecomastia, liver dysfunction, but IM testosterone is inexpensive and generally well tolerated

Table 74. Management of Male Sexual Dysfunction (cont.)		
Cause	Therapy	Comments
	or testosterone gel 1% (*AndroGel*) [5 g (50 mg/24 h), 7.5 g (75 mg), 10 g (100 mg)] begin with 5 g pk qam	Squeeze pk contents into palm of hand and apply, let dry; wash hands immediately. Check serum testosterone after 14 d and adjust dose; do not use in women.
Neuropathic, vascular, or mixed	Vacuum tumescence devices (*Osbon-Erec Aid, Catalyst Vacuum Device, Pos-T-Vac, Rejoyn*)	Rare: Ecchymosis, reduced ejaculation, coolness of penile tip. Good acceptance in older population; intercourse successful in 70% to 90% of cases
	Intracavernosal [5, 10, 20, 40 μg] *or* intraurethral [125, 250, 500, 1000 μg] prostaglandin E (*Alprostadil*)	Risks: hypotension, bruising, bleeding, priapism; erection > 4 h requires emergency treatment; intraurethral safer and more acceptable
	Penile prosthesis	Complications: infection, mechanical failure, penile fibrosis
Organic, psychogenic, or mixed	Sildenafil (*Viagra*) [25, 50, 100] start 25 mg 1 h before sexual activity; maximum 1/d Vardenafil (*Levitra*) [2.5, 5, 10, 20] 5 mg 1 h before sexual activity	Contraindicated with use of nitrates; contraindicated with use of α-blockers (vardenafil); caution in vascular disease; least effective in vascular impotence. Several other drug interactions; metabolism reduced in liver and kidney disease, and aging. Side effects: headache, flushing, dyspepsia (mild and transient), color tinge in vision (sildenafil), nasal congestion, UTI, diarrhea, dizziness, and rash

DYSPAREUNIA
Definition
Pain with intercourse.

Aggravating Factors
- Gynecologic tumors
- Interstitial cystitis
- Myalgia from overexertion during Kegel's exercises
- Osteroarthritis
- Pelvic fractures
- Retroverted uterus
- Sacral nerve root compression
- Vaginal atrophy from estrogen deprivation
- Vulvar or vaginal infection

Evaluation
- Ask about sexual problems (eg, changes in libido, partner's function, and health issues).
- Screen for depression.
- Perform pelvic examination for vulvovaginitis, vaginal atrophy, conization (decreased distensibility and narrowing of the vaginal canal), scarring, pelvic inflammatory disease, cystocele, and rectocele.

Management
- Identify and treat clinical pathology.
- Educate and counsel patients.
- Discuss hormone therapy (see pp 180–182).
- Water-soluble lubricants (eg, *Replens*) are highly effective as monotherapy for those who cannot or will not use hormones, or as a supplement to estrogen.
- For vaginismus (vaginal muscle spasm), trial cessation of intercourse and gradual vaginal dilation may help.
- For diminished libido, short-term use of androgens (which used long-term adversely affect health) may help; refer for counseling or sex therapy.
- For atrophic vaginitis: estrogen cream, use minimum dose (eg, 0.5 g *Premarin* [42.5 g], 2 g *Ogen* or *Estrace* [42.5 g]), daily for 2 wk, then 1–3 × /wk thereafter; estradiol vaginal ring (*Estring*) inserted intravaginally and changed q 90 d, high degree of safety and acceptability; estradiol vaginal tablets (*Vagifem* 25 μg) inserted intravaginally daily × 2 wk, then twice/wk.

SSRI-INDUCED SEXUAL DYSFUNCTION
- Incidence varies widely, from 1% to 20% of patients making spontaneous reports to 75% when patients are systematically questioned.
- Symptoms include anorgasmia, decreased libido, and ejaculatory dysfunction.
- Tolerance may develop up to 12 wk on treatment.
- Pharmacologic management:
  - For sertraline and citalopram (not other SSRIs), reducing dose or drug holidays (skip or reduce weekend dose) may help.
  - Adjuvant medications reported as effective for this condition in case reports include
    - Bupropion (*Wellbutrin SR, Zyban*) 75–100 mg po qd
    - Mirtazapine (*Remeron*) 15 mg po hs
    - Sildenafil (*Viagra*) 25–100 mg 1 h before intercourse
- Controlled trials of mirtazapine, yohimbine, olanzapine, and bupropion failed to show a benefit different from that of placebo, although most trials were small.

CHRONIC WOUND ASSESSMENT AND TREATMENT
Wound Assessment
Evaluation of chronic wounds should include the following (see **Table 75** for wound characteristics specific to ulcer type):
- Location
- Wound size and shape: length, width, depth, stage (pressure ulcer), grade (diabetic foot ulcer)
- Wound bed: color, presence of slough, necrotic tissue, granulation tissue, epithelial tissue, undermining or tunneling
- Exudate: purulent vs nonpurulent (serous, serosanguineous)
- Wound edges: distinct, diffuse, rolled under
- Periwound surface: erythema, edema, induration, temperature
- Presence of pain
- Signs of wound infection
  - Increased necrotic tissue
  - Foul odor of exudates
  - Purulent exudates
  - Faint halo of erythema at wound edges
  - Wound breakdown
  - Increasing pain
  - Edema
  - Granulation tissue that bleeds easily
  - Serous exudates with inflammation
  - Nonhealing or enlarging wound
  - Swab culture of limited value in diagnosing infection due to contaminated wound bed

Wound Treatment
- Remove devitalized tissues and surface contaminants
  - Sharp debridement
  - Autolytic enzymatic preparations (eg, moisture-retaining dressings or hydrogels)
  - Mechanical (eg, wet-to-dry dressings)
  - Chemical (eg, topical enzymes such as *Accuzyme, Santyl*)
  - Cleanse with irrigation or whirlpool using normal saline or lactated Ringer's solution
  - Avoid antiseptics due to cytotoxicity
- Control bacterial burden of wound
  - Monitor for signs of infection
  - Debride all necrotic tissue
  - Limit use of topical antibiotics due to risk of developing resistant organisms
  - Use systemic antibiotics only in presence of spreading cellulitis, sepsis, or osteomyelitis
- Provide moist wound environment and control exudates with dressings (see **Table 76** and **Table 77**)
- Prevent further injury
  - Position to avoid any pressure on the wound
- Support repair process
  - Protein and calories (protein: 1.25–1.5 g/kg/d; calories: 30–35 calories/kg/d)
  - Vitamin and mineral supplements if deficiencies suspected
  - Avoid exposure to cold; vasoconstriction reduces blood flow to wound

Table 75. Wound Characteristics by Ulcer Etiology				
	Arterial	**Diabetic**	**Pressure**	**Venous**
Location	Tips of toes or between toes, on pressure points of foot (eg, heel or lateral foot), or in areas of trauma	Plantar surface of foot, especially over metatarsal heads, toes, and heel	Over bony prominences (eg, trochanter, coccyx, ankle)	Gaiter area, particularly medial malleolus
Size and shape	Small craters with well-defined borders	Even wound margins with callus	Variable length, width, depth depending on stage (see staging system, p 163)	Edges may be irregular with depth limited to dermis or shallow subcutaneous tissue
Wound bed	Pale or necrotic	Granular tissue unless PAD present	Varies from bright red, shallow crater to deeper crater with slough and necrotic tissue; tunneling and undermining	Ruddy red; yellow slough may be present; undermining or tunneling uncommon
Exudate	Minimal amount due to poor blood flow	Variable amount; serous unless infection present	Purulent, becoming serous as healing progresses; foul odor with infection	Copious; serous unless infection present
Surrounding skin	Halo of erythema or slight fluctuance indicative of infection	Normal	May be distinct, diffuse, rolled under; erythema, edema, induration if infected	May appear macerated, crusted, or scaling
Pain	Cramping or constant deep aching	None due to neuropathy	Painful, unless sensory function impaired	Variable; may be severe, dull, aching, or bursting in character

ARTERIAL ULCERS
Definition
Any lesion caused by severe tissue ischemia secondary to atherosclerosis.

Etiologic Factors for Arterial Ulcer Development
- Progressive occlusion
- Minor trauma (eg, footwear)

Intrinsic Risk Factors
- Peripheral arterial disease (PAD)
- Diabetes mellitus
- Systolic hypertension
- Smoking
- Advanced age

Evaluation

In addition to evaluation under Chronic Wound Assessment (see p 157):

- Determine severity of PAD (see p 37)
  - Venous filling time: Prolonged venous filling (>20 sec) predictive of severe PAD
  - Pedal pulses: Absence of both a dorsalis pedis and a posterior tibialis pulse indicative of PAD
  - Skin temperature: Unilateral coolness and sudden, marked change from proximal to distal
  - Ankle-brachial index: If ABI value < 0.5, wound healing unlikely without revascularization
- Assess wound characteristics (see **Table 75**)
- Assess pain characteristics (see Pain, p 119)

Prevention and Management

Protective Skin Care:
- Inspect feet and legs daily
- Use emollients after bathing to prevent cracking and fissures
- Dry skin between toes to prevent maceration
- Avoid friction and pressure by using lamb's wool or foam between toes
- Use positioning devices to avoid pressure on feet (eg, heel protectors)

Protection from Mechanical Trauma:
- Wear proper fitting, protective footwear consistently
- Seek professional foot and nail care

Protection from Thermal Trauma:
- Wear warm socks to prevent vasoconstriction
- Avoid exposure of feet and legs to heat-producing devices and hot bathing water

Local Wound Care

Treatment dictated by adequacy of perfusion and status of wound bed:

- Avoid debridement of necrotic tissue until perfusion status is determined.
- If wound is infected, revascularization procedures, surgical removal of necrotic tissue, and systemic antibiotics are treatments of choice.
- Topical antibiotics should not be relied on to treat infected ischemic wounds and may cause sensitivity reactions.
- If wound is uninfected and dry eschar is present, maintain dry intact eschar as a barrier to bacteria. Application of an antiseptic may decrease bacterial burden on wound surface.
- If wound is uninfected and soft slough and necrotic tissue is present, apply moisture-retaining dressings that allow frequent inspection of wound for signs of infection.
- Assess vascular perfusion and refer for surgical intervention if consistent with overall goals of care.

DIABETIC FOOT ULCERS

Definition

Any lesion on the plantar surface of the foot caused by neuropathy.

Etiologic Factors for Diabetic Ulcer Development

Repetitive stress, unrelieved pressure and trauma in an insensate foot

Intrinsic Risk Factors

- Peripheral neuropathy
- Structural foot deformity
- Limited joint mobility
- History of previous ulcers
- History of amputation
- Retinopathy
- Nephropathy
- History of uncontrolled or poorly controlled diabetes
- Advanced age
- Vascular insufficiency
- Poorly fitting footwear

Evaluation

In addition to evaluation under Chronic Wound Assessment (see p 157):
- Assess the feet in patients with one or more risk factors:
  - Visual inspection for rubor, pallor, callus, dry skin, ingrown toenails, and fissures
  - Vascular assessment for pulses, dorsal vein distention, temperature
  - Sensory assessment for pressure, touch, vibration
  - Motor assessment for joint rigidity, muscle wasting, gait disturbance
- Assess wound characteristics (see **Table 75**)
- Assess for presence of infection:
  - Sudden increase in blood glucose
  - Wound can be probed to the bone—highly sensitive indicator of osteomyelitis
- Determine grade of ulcer (Wagner Classification)
  - Grade 0: Preulcerative lesions; healed ulcers present; bony deformity present
  - Grade 1: Superficial ulcer without subcutaneous tissue involvement
  - Grade 2: Penetration through subcutaneous tissue
  - Grade 3: Ostitis, abscess, or osteomyelitis
  - Grade 4: Gangrene of digit
  - Grade 5: Gangrene of foot requiring disarticulation

Prevention and Management

- Inspect feet daily
- Use emollients after bathing to prevent cracking and fissures
- Wear proper fitting, protective footwear consistently
- Seek professional foot and nail care
- Avoid exposure to heat-producing devices (eg, heating pads) and hot bathing water

Local Wound Care

In addition to recommendations under Chronic Wound Treatment (see p 157):
- Debride devitalized tissue and callus: surgical debridement is method of choice for effective, rapid removal of nonviable tissue
- Avoid occlusive dressings due to risk of wound infection

- Offload pressure and stress from foot
  - Avoidance of pressure on foot essential to management of diabetic foot ulcer
  - Use orthotic that redistributes weight on plantar surface of foot when ambulating (eg, total contact cast, *DH Pressure Relief™ Walker*)
- Topical antibiotics should not be relied on to treat diabetic foot ulcer infections due to development of resistant organisms.

Pharmacologic Therapy
- *Regranex®*, a recombinant platelet-derived growth factor, applied topically in thin layer to a clean wound bed for 12 h followed by 12 h of saline-moistened gauze dressing
  - Must be used in conjunction with offloading of pressure on foot, regular sharp debridement, and maintenance of uninfected status.
  - If 30% wound closure has not occurred in 10 wk or complete closure in 20 wk, reevaluate treatment plan and consider surgical intervention (especially if osteomyelitis is present).
  - Monitor healing progress; if no signs of healing over 2-wk period, reevaluate factors affecting healing and wound management strategies.

Surgical Intervention
- If ulceration is resistant to more conservative therapies or if osteomyelitis is suspected, referral for surgical evaluation is warranted.

PRESSURE ULCERS
Definition
Any lesion caused by unrelieved pressure resulting in damage of underlying tissue; usually occurs over bony prominence.

Etiologic Factors for Pressure Ulcer Development
- Pressure
- Shear
- Friction

Intrinsic Risk Factors
- Immobility (eg, chairbound)
- Increased age
- Malnutrition
- Moisture (eg, incontinence)
- Decreased sensory perception

Table 76. Wound and Pressure Ulcer Products, by Drainage and Stage							
		Drainage			Wound Stage		
Product	Light	Moderate	Heavy	I	II	III	IV
Transparent film	•			•	•		
Foam island		•			•	•	
Hydrocolloids	•	•			•	•	
Petroleum-based nonadherent	•				•	•	
Alginate		•	•			•	•
Hydrogel	•				•	•	•
Gauze packing (moistened with saline)		•	•			•	•

Table 77. Common Dressings for Pressure Ulcer Treatment			
Dressing	**Indications**	**Contraindications**	**Examples**
Transparent film	Stage I, II Protection from friction Superficial scrape Autolytic debridement of slough Apply skin prep to intact skin to protect from adhesive	Draining ulcers Suspicion of skin infection or fungus	*Bioclusive* *Tegaderm* *Op-site*
Foam island	Stage II, III Low to moderate exudate Can apply as window to secure transparent film	Excessive exudate Dry, crusted wound	*Alleyn* *Lyofoam*
Hydrocolloids	Stage II, III Low to moderate drainage Good peri-wound skin integrity Autolytic debridement of slough Left in place 3–5 d Can apply as window to secure transparent film Can apply over alginate to control drainage Must control maceration Apply skin prep to intact skin to protect from adhesive	Poor skin integrity Infected ulcers Wound needs packing	*DuoDerm* *Extra thin film DuoDerm* *Tegasorb* *RepliCare* *Comfel* *Nu-derm*
Alginate	Stage III, IV Excessive drainage Apply dressing within wound borders Requires secondary dressing Must use skin prep Must control for maceration	Dry or minimally draining wound Superficial wounds with maceration	*Sorbsan* *Kaltostet* *Algosteril* *AlgiDerm*
Hydrogel (amorphous gels)	Stage II, III, IV Needs to be combined with gauze dressing Stays moist longer than saline gauze Changed 1–2 times/d Used as alternative to saline gauze for packing deep wounds with tunnels, undermining Reduces adherence of gauze to wound Must control for maceration	Macerated areas Wounds with excess exudate	*IntraSite gel* *Solosite gel* *Restore gel*
(gel sheet)	Stage II Needs to be held in place with topper dressing	Macerated areas Wounds with moderate to heavy exudate	*Vigilon* *Restore Impregnated Gauze*
Gauze packing (moistened with saline)	Stage III, IV Wounds with depth, especially those with tunnels, undermining Must be remoistened often to maintain moist wound environment		Square 2 × 2s, 4 × 4s *Fluffed Kerlix* *Plain Nugauze*

Source: Copyright © 2004 by Rita Frantz. Used with permission.

Evaluation

In addition to evaluation under Chronic Wound Assessment (see p 157):

- Determine intensity of risk status using validated tool, eg, Braden Scale; see Braden BJ, Bergstrom N. Clinical utility of the Braden Scale for predicting pressure sore risk. *Decubitus* 1989;2(3):44–51; for online versions of the scale: www.skinwound.com/online_training_manual/braden_scale.htm (for a downloadable PDF file)
http://text.nlm.nih.gov (in AHRQ pressure ulcer practice guideline).
- Assess wound characteristics (see **Table 75** and below)
- Determine level of tissue injury by using Pressure Ulcer Staging System:
  - **Stage I:** An observable pressure-related alteration of intact skin whose indicators as compared with an adjacent or opposite area on the body may include changes in one or more of the following: skin temperature (warmth or coolness), tissue consistency (firm or boggy feel), and/or sensation (pain, itching). The ulcer appears as a defined area of persistent redness in lightly pigmented skin, whereas in darker skin tones, it may appear with persistent red, blue, or purple hues.
  - **Stage II:** Partial-thickness skin loss involving epidermis and/or dermis; presents as abrasion, blister, or shallow crater.
  - **Stage III:** Full-thickness skin loss involving damage or necrosis of subcutaneous tissue that may extend down to, but not through, underlying fascia; presents as deep crater with or without undermining of adjacent tissue.
  - **Stage IV:** Full-thickness skin loss with extensive destruction, tissue necrosis, or damage to muscle, bone, or supporting structures. May have associated undermining of sinus tracts. Note: eschar-covered ulcers cannot be staged until eschar is removed.

Prevention and Management

In addition to recommendations under Chronic Wound Treatment (see p 157):
Protect Wound and Surrounding Skin from Further Trauma
- Avoid positioning directly on the ulcer.
- Employ pressure-reduction strategies:
  - Reposition every 2 h.
  - Use pressure-reducing cushions, mattresses, and heel protectors.
  - Avoid massaging reddened bony prominences.
  - Avoid positioning directly on the trochanter.
- Reduce friction and shear:
  - Maintain head of bed elevation < 30 degrees.
  - Use lift sheet to reposition.
Promote Clean Wound Bed, Prevent Infection
- Debride necrotic tissue, eschar
- Autolytic methods or topical enzymes may be used in conjunction with sharp debridement to facilitate more rapid removal of necrotic tissue.
- Cleanse with each dressing change using normal saline. Irrigate using 8 mm Hg pressure (19-gauge IV catheter and 35-cc syringe) when wound is deep, tunneled, or undermined.

Maintain Moist Wound Environment (See **Table 76** and **Table 77**)

Control Exudate (See **Table 76** and **Table 77**)

Eliminate Dead Space
• Pack dead space (tunnels, undermining) with moistened gauze dressings or strips of calcium alginate

Diagnose and Treat Infection
• Ensure that necrotic tissue has been debrided completely from wound bed.
• Consider 2-wk trial of topical antibiotic for clean ulcers that are not healing after 2–4 wk optimal care; antibiotic should be effective against gram-negative, gram-positive, and anaerobic organisms.
• Avoid using systemic antibiotics in the absence of advancing cellulitis or systemic infection.

Support Healing Systemically
• Provide nutritional support (see p 92)
• Provide adequate hydration with oral or parenteral fluids

Surgical Repair
• Consider surgical referral for Stage IV pressure ulcers and for severely undermined or tunneled wounds
• Monitor healing progress; in absence of signs of healing over 2-wk period, reevaluate factors affecting healing and wound management strategies

VENOUS ULCERS
Definition
Any lesion caused by venous insufficiency precipitated by venous hypertension.

Etiologic Factors for Venous Ulcer Development
• Venous insufficiency

Intrinsic Risk Factors
• Deep vein thrombosis
• Multiple pregnancies
• Edema
• Ascites
• Congenital anomalies
• Severe trauma to legs
• Tumors
• Sedentary lifestyle or job

Evaluation
In addition to evaluation under Chronic Wound Assessment (see p 157):
• Assess status of venous insufficiency
  - Lower extremity edema
  - Lipodermatosclerosis (hyperpigmentation and induration around gaiter area)
  - Varicosities
  - Hemosiderosis
  - Venous dermatitis
• Diagnostic studies: Doppler ultrasonography, duplex imaging
• Assess wound characteristics (see **Table 75**)

Prevention and Management
Compression Therapy:
- Essential component of venous ulcer treatment
- Provides externally applied pressure or static support to lower extremity to facilitate normal venous return
- Therapeutic level of compression is 30–40 mm Hg at the ankle, decreasing toward the knee
- Contraindicated in arterial insufficiency, uncompensated congestive heart failure and active thrombus
- Avoid compression therapy when ABI < 0.8
- Types of compression therapy:
  - Static compression
    - Therapeutic stockings
      - Use with stable venous insufficiency to prevent ulceration or with an existing ulcer once edema has been controlled.
    - Compression wraps
      - Combination short- and long-stretch elastic wraps (eg, *Dynaflex, Profore*) provide sustained compression for ambulatory or sedentary patient
      - Avoid long-stretch elastic wraps (eg, *Ace* bandages, antiembolism hose) that provide sub-therapeutic levels of compression
      - Inelastic devices (paste bandages and orthotic devices (eg, *Unna's boot, Circ-Aid Thera-Boot*) work by compressing calf during ambulation; most effective for ambulatory patients
  - Dynamic compression: Powered devices that propel venous blood upward when applied to lower extremity (eg, intermittent pneumatic pumps, sequential gradient compression devices, A-V impulse device)

Local Wound Care
In addition to recommendations under Chronic Wound Treatment (see p 157):
- Use exudate-absorbing dressings (eg, calcium alginate dressings, foam dressings)
- Use skin sealant to protect skin around wound from exudates
- Topical antibiotics should not be relied on to treat venous ulcer infections due to development of resistant organisms.

Pharmacologic Therapy
- Pentoxifylline (*Trental*) 400–800 mg tid has been shown to accelerate healing by decreasing blood viscosity and WBC adhesion while increasing fibrinolysis.

Surgical Intervention
- If manifestations of chronic venous insufficiency and ulceration are resistant to more conservative therapies or if venous obstruction is present, surgical repair (eg, skin graft) is treatment of choice.
- Monitor healing progress; if no signs of healing over 2-wk period, reevaluate factors affecting healing and wound management strategies.

SLEEP DISORDERS

CLASSIFICATION
- Disturbance of the sleep-wake cycle
- Hypersomnolence
- Insomnia (difficulty initiating or maintaining sleep)
- Parasomnias (disorders of arousal, partial arousal, and sleep stage transition)
- Sleep apnea

SLEEP DISORDERS OTHER THAN SLEEP APNEA
Risk Factors and Aggravating Factors
Treatable Associated Medical and Psychiatric Conditions: Adjustment disorders, anxiety, bereavement, cough, depression, dyspnea (cardiac or pulmonary), GERD, nocturia, pain, paresthesias, stress
Medications That Cause or Aggravate Sleep Problems: Alcohol, antidepressants, β-blockers, bronchodilators, caffeine, clonidine, cortisone, diuretics, levodopa, methyldopa, nicotine, phenytoin, progesterone, quinidine, reserpine, sedatives, sympathomimetics including decongestants

Management
Sleep improvements are better sustained over time with behavioral treatment.
Nonpharmacologic—Measures Recommended to Improve Sleep Hygiene:
- During the daytime:
  - Get out of bed at the same time each morning regardless of how much you slept the night before.
  - Exercise daily, but not immediately before bedtime.
  - Get adequate exposure to bright light during the day.
  - Decrease or eliminate naps, unless necessary part of sleeping schedule.
  - Limit or eliminate alcohol, caffeine, and nicotine, especially before bedtime.
- At bedtime:
  - Maintain a regular sleeping time, but don't go to bed unless sleepy.
  - If hungry, have a light snack before bed (unless there are symptoms of GERD or it is otherwise medically contraindicated), but avoid heavy meals at bedtime.
  - Don't read or watch television in bed.
  - Relax mentally before going to sleep; don't use bedtime as worry time.
  - Relax before bedtime, and maintain a routine period of preparation for bed (eg, washing up and going to the bathroom).
  - Control the nighttime environment with comfortable temperature, quietness, darkness.
  - Wear comfortable bedclothes.
  - If it helps, use soothing noise, for example, a fan or other appliance or a "white noise" machine.
  - If unable to fall asleep within 15–20 min, get out of bed and perform soothing activity, such as listening to soft music or reading (but avoid exposure to bright light during these times).

Pharmacologic—Principles of Prescribing Medications for Sleep Disorders:

- Use lowest effective dose.
- Use intermittent dosing (2–4 times/wk).
- Prescribe medications for short-term use (no more than 3–4 wk).
- Discontinue medication gradually.
- Be alert for rebound insomnia following discontinuation.

Table 78. Useful Medications for Sleep Disorders in Elderly Persons				
Class, Drug	Usual Dose	Formulations	Half-Life	Comments (Metabolism, Excretion)
Antidepressant, sedating				
√ Trazodone (*Desyrel*)	25–150 mg	T: 50, 100, 150, 300	12 h	Moderate orthostatic effects; effective for insomnia with or without depression (L)
Benzodiazepine, intermediate-acting				
Estazolam (*ProSom*)	0.5–1.0 mg	T: 1, 2	12–18 h	Rapidly absorbed, effective in initiating sleep; slightly active metabolites that may accumulate (K)
Lorazepam (*Ativan*)	0.25–2 mg	T: 0.5, 1, 2	8–12 h	Effective in initiating and maintaining sleep; associated with falls, memory loss, rebound insomnia (K)
Temazepam (*Restoril*)	7.5–15 mg	C: 7.5, 15, 30	8–10 h*	Daytime drowsiness may occur with repeated use; effective for sleep maintenance; delayed onset of effect (K)
Nonbenzodiazepine, short-acting				
Zaleplon (*Sonata*)	5 mg	C: 5, 10	1 h	Avoid taking with alcohol or food (L)
Zolpidem (*Ambien*)	5 mg	T: 5, 10	1.5–4.5 h**	Confusion and agitation may occur but are rare (L)
CNS depressant, nonbarbiturate and nonbenzodiazepine				
Chloral hydrate (*Aquachloral, Supprettes*)	500–1000 mg (not to exceed 2 g as single dose or total daily dose)	C: 500; syr 500 mg/ 5 mL; Sp: 324, 500, 648	8 h (active metabo- lite)	Hypnotic effect lost after 2 wk of continuous use; contraindicated in marked cardiac, hepatic, or renal impairment (K, L)
Hormone				
Melatonin	0.3–5 mg	various	1 h	Not regulated by FDA

√ = preferred for treating older persons.
* Can be as long as 30 h in elderly persons.
** 3 h in elderly persons; 10 h in those with hepatic cirrhosis.

SLEEP APNEA

Definition

Repeated episodes of apnea (cessation of airflow for ≥ 10 sec) or hypopnea (transient reduction [≥ 30% decrease in thoracoabdominal movement or airflow and with at least 4% oxygen desaturation or an arousal] of airflow for ≥ 10 sec) during sleep with excessive daytime sleepiness or altered cardiopulmonary function.

Classification

Obstructive (90% of cases): Airflow cessation as a result of upper airway closure in spite of adequate respiratory muscle effort
Central: Cessation of respiratory effort
Mixed: Features of both obstructive and central

Associated Risk Factors, Clinical Features

Family hx, HTN, increased neck circumference, male gender, obesity, smoking, snoring, upper airway structural abnormalities (eg, soft palate, tonsils)

Evaluation

- Full night's sleep study (polysomnography) in sleep laboratory indicated for those who habitually snore and either report daytime sleepiness or have observed apnea.
- Results are reported as the apnea-hypopnea index (AHI), which is the number of episodes of apneas and hypopneas per hour of sleep.
- Threshold for CPAP reimbursement by Medicare based on a minimum of 2 h sleep by polysomnography is AHI (1) ≥ 15 or (2) ≥ 5 and ≤ 14 with documented symptoms of excessive daytime sleepiness, impaired cognition, mood disorders, or insomnia, or documented HTN, ischemic heart disease, or hx of stroke.

Management

Nonpharmacologic:
- Use CPAP by nasal mask, nasal prongs, or mask that covers the nose and mouth (considered initial treatment for clinically important sleep apnea).
- Avoid use of alcohol or sedatives.
- Lie in lateral rather than supine position; may be facilitated by soft foam ball in a backpack.
- Lose weight (obese patients).
- Use oral appliances that keep the tongue in an anterior position during sleep or keep the mandible forward.

Pharmacologic: Beneficial mostly in mild sleep apnea.
- Protriptyline (*Vivactil*) 10–20 mg/d [T: 5, 10] L (men commonly experience urinary hesitancy or frequency and impotence)
- Fluoxetine (*Prozac*) 10–20 mg [T: 10, 20, 40; S: 20 mg/5 mL] L

Surgical:
- Tracheostomy (indicated for patients with severe apnea who cannot tolerate positive pressure or when other interventions are ineffective)
- Uvulopalatopharyngoplasty (curative in fewer than 50% of cases)
- Maxillofacial surgery (rare cases)

OTHER CONDITIONS ASSOCIATED WITH SLEEP DISORDERS
Nocturnal Leg Cramps
Stretching exercises may be helpful. Quinine, 200–300 mg po hs [T: 200, 260, 300, 325] may reduce the frequency though not the severity of leg cramps. Cinchonism, hemolysis, thrombocytopenia, and visual disturbances are notable side effects.

Restless Legs Syndrome
Diagnostic Criteria:
- A compelling urge to move the limbs, usually associated with paresthesias/dysasthesias
- Motor restlessness (eg, floor pacing, tossing and turning in bed, rubbing legs)
- Vague discomfort, usually bilateral, most commonly in calves
- Symptoms exacerbated by rest, especially at night
- Symptoms relieved by movement—jerking, stretching, or shaking of limbs; pacing

Secondary Causes: iron deficiency, spinal cord and peripheral nerve lesions, uremia, drugs (eg, TCAs, SSRIs, lithium, dopamine antagonists, caffeine)

Nonpharmacologic Treatment:
- Sleep hygiene measures (see p 166)
- Avoid alcohol, caffeine, nicotine.
- Rub limbs.
- Use hot or cold baths, whirlpools.

Pharmacologic Treatment
- Exclude or treat iron deficiency, peripheral neuropathy.
- If possible, avoid SSRIs, TCAs, lithium, and dopamine antagonists.

Start at low dose, increase as needed:
- First line: dopamine agonists (see **Table 54**) or carbidopa-levodopa (*Sinemet*) 25/100 mg, 1–2 h before bedtime. Patients may develop symptom augmentation that occurs earlier in the day (eg, afternoon instead of evening) and may be more severe. Treatment of augmentation may require reduction of dose or switch to dopamine agonist.
- Second-line agents include carbamazepine and gabapentin (see **Table 55**).
- For refractory cases, benzodiazepines or opioids can be tried.

Periodic Limb Movement Disorder
Diagnostic Criteria:
- Insomnia or excessive sleepiness
- Repetitive, highly stereotyped limb muscle movements (eg, extension of big toes with partial flexion of ankle, knee, and sometimes hip)
- Polysomnographic monitoring showing repetitive episodes of muscle contractions and associated arousals or awakenings
- No evidence of a medical, mental, or other sleep disorder that can account for symptoms

Treatment: Indicated for clinically significant sleep disruption or frequent arousals documented on a sleep study.
- Nonpharmacologic: sleep hygiene measures (see p 166)
- Pharmacologic: See restless legs syndrome, above.

GENERAL INFORMATION

UI is not a normal part of aging. It is a loss of urine control due to a combination of
- Genitourinary pathology
- Age-related changes
- Comorbid conditions
- Environmental obstacles

CLASSIFICATION

Reversible Causes of Incontinence (DRIP Mnemonic)

Delirium
Restricted mobility (illness, injury, gait disorder, restraint)
Infection (acute, symptomatic); **I**nflammation (atrophic vaginitis); **I**mpaction of stool
Polyuria (diabetes mellitus, caffeine intake, volume overload); **P**harmaceuticals (diuretics, autonomic agents, psychotropics)

Established Incontinence

Urge: Detrusor muscle overactivity (uninhibited bladder contractions); small to large volume loss; may be idiopathic or associated with CNS lesions or bladder irritation from infection, stones, tumors; may be associated with impaired contractility and retention (detrusor hyperactivity with impaired contractility [DHIC]).

Stress: Failure of sphincter mechanisms to remain closed during bladder filling (often due to insufficient pelvic support in women and trauma from prostate surgery in men); loss occurs with increased intra-abdominal pressure.

Overflow: Impaired detrusor contractility or bladder outlet obstruction. Impaired contractility—chronic outlet obstruction, diabetes mellitus, vitamin B_{12} deficiency, tabes dorsalis, alcoholism, or spinal disease. Outlet obstruction—in men, BPH, cancer, stricture; in women, prior incontinence surgery or large cystocele.

Mixed: Combined urge and stress UI is common in older women.

Functional: Inability or unwillingness to toilet because of physical, cognitive, psychologic, or environmental factors.

Other (Rare): Bladder-sphincter dyssynergia, fistulas, reduced detrusor compliance, recurrent cystitis.

RISK FACTORS

- Age-related changes (BPH, atrophic urethritis)
- Constipation
- Dementia, depression, stroke, Parkinson's disease
- Detrusor overactivity and uninhibited contractions
- Fecal incontinence
- HF, nocturia, COPD, or chronic cough
- Increased postvoid residual or decreased bladder capacity
- Impaired ADLs
- Obesity

EVALUATION
History
- Precipitant urgency suggests detrusor overactivity.
- Loss with cough, laugh, or bend suggests stress.
- Continuous leakage suggests intrinsic sphincter insufficiency or overflow.
- Onset, frequency, volume, timing, precipitants (eg, caffeine, diuretics, alcohol, cough, medications).

Physical Examination
- Functional status (eg, mobility, dexterity)
- Mental status
- Orthostatic BP, HR
- Findings:
  - Bladder distension
  - Cervical cord compression (interosseus muscle wasting, Hoffmann's or Babinski's signs)
  - Rectal mass or impaction
  - Sacral root integrity (anal sphincter tone, anal wink, perineal sensation)
  - Volume overload, edema

Male GU
Prostate consistency; symmetry; for uncircumcised, check phimosis, paraphimosis, balanitis

Female GU
Atrophic vaginitis (see p 156 for treatment); pelvic support (see ACOG classification, p 180)

Testing
Voiding Record: Record time and volume of incontinent, continent episodes; activities and time of sleep; knowing oral intake is sometimes helpful.
Standing Full Bladder Stress Test: Relax perineum and cough once—immediate loss suggests stress, several seconds' delay suggests detrusor overactivity.
Postvoid Residual: If > 100 mL, repeat; still > 100 mL suggests detrusor weakness, neuropathy, outlet obstruction, or DHIC.
Laboratory: UA and urine C&S; glucose and calcium if polyuric; renal function tests and B_{12} if urinary retention; urine cytology if hematuria or pain; PSA if cancer suspected.
Urodynamic Testing: Not routinely indicated; indicated before corrective surgery, when diagnosis is unclear, or when empiric therapy fails.

MANAGEMENT
In a stepped approach, treat all transient causes first (DRIP); avoid caffeine, alcohol, minimize evening intake of fluids.

Nonpharmacologic Behavioral Therapy (First-Line Therapy)
Detrusor Instability: Timed toileting—shortest interval to keep dry; urge control—when urgency occurs, sit or stand quietly, focus on letting urge pass, when no longer urgent walk slowly to the bathroom and void. When no incontinence for 2 d, increase voiding

interval by 30–60 min until voiding every 3–4 h. Electrical stimulation often effective; refer to PT. Pelvic muscle exercises (see below).

Cognitively Impaired Persons: Prompted toileting (ask if patient needs to void) at 2- to 3-h intervals during day; encourage patients to report continence status; praise patient when continent and responds to toileting.

Stress Incontinence: Pelvic muscle (Kegel's) exercises—isolate pelvic muscles (avoid thigh, rectal, buttocks contraction); perform 3–10 sets of 10 contractions at maximum strength daily; progressively longer (up to 10-sec) contractions; follow-up and encouragement necessary; consider biofeedback for training or have patient practice interrupting urine stream while voiding.

Pessaries: May benefit women with vaginal or uterine prolapse.

Detrusor Hyperactivity with Impaired Contractility: Treat urge first; self-intermittent clean catheterization if needed.

Pharmacologic Therapy

Estrogen replacement benefits urge and possibly stress UI; see **Table 83** for recommended dose regimens. Topical estrogens are also effective; see p 156 for available preparations. See **Table 79** for other therapies.

Table 79. Drugs to Treat Urinary Incontinence, by Types			
R$_x$ by UI Type	Dosage	Formulations	Comments (Metabolism)
Urge or Mixed UI*			
Dicyclomine (*Bentyl*)	10–20 mg tid	T: 20; C: 10; S: syr 10 mg/5 mL	Dry mouth, blurry vision, ↑ intraocular pressure, delirium, constipation, plus postural ↓ BP, cardiac conduction disturbances (K)
Hyoscyamine (*Anaspaz, Cystospaz, Levsin*)	0.375–0.75 mg qid 0.375–0.75 po q 12 h	T: 0.125; S: elixir 0.125 mg/5 mL SR: 0.375	May exhibit less dry mouth, depending on dosage; delirium, nervousness, insomnia (K)
Imipramine (*Tofranil*)	10–50 mg qd	T: 10, 25, 50	Dry mouth, blurry vision, ↑ intraocular pressure, delirium, constipation, plus postural ↓ BP, cardiac conduction disturbances (L)
√ Oxybutynin (*Ditropan, Ditropan XL, Oxytrol*)	2.5–5.0 mg bid–tid 5–20 mg qd 3.9 mg/d (apply patch 2 × /wk)	T: 5; S: 5 mg/ 5 mL SR: 5, 10, 15 transdermal 39 cm² patch	Dry mouth, blurry vision, ↑ intraocular pressure, delirium, constipation (L) No more dry mouth than placebo; may irritate skin
Propantheline (*Pro-Banthine*)	15–30 mg tid (on empty stomach)	T: 15	Dry mouth, blurry vision, ↑ intraocular pressure, delirium, constipation (L, K)
Flavoxate (*Urispas*)	100–200 mg tid–qid	T: 100	Tachycardia, palpitations, drowsiness, delirium, nausea, vomiting, dry mouth, ↑ intraocular pressure (L, K)
√ Tolterodine (*Detrol, Detrol LA*)	2 mg bid 4 mg qd	T: 1, 2 C: ER 2, 4	Dry mouth, dyspepsia, constipation, delirium (L)

Table 79. Drugs to Treat Urinary Incontinence, by Types (cont.)			
R_x by UI Type	Dosage	Formulations	Comments (Metabolism)
Stress UI[†]			
Pseudoephedrine (eg, *Sudafed*)	15–30 mg tid	T: 30, 60; elixir 30 mg/5 mL	Headache, tachycardia, ↑ BP (L)
(*Sudafed XR*)	120 mg qd, bid	SR: 120	

Note: √ = preferred in treating older people. For prostate obstruction UI, see p 141.
*Drugs to treat urge or mixed UI: ↑ bladder capacity, ↓ involuntary contractions.
[†]Drugs to treat stress UI: ↑ urethral smooth muscle contraction.

Surgical Therapy
• Consider for the 50% of women whose stress UI does not respond adequately to behavioral treatment and exercise.
• Urinary sphincter function has proximal, distal, and intrinsic components; a surgical approach addresses only one component.
  - Traditional surgery (retropubic colposuspension) addresses the proximal defect.
  - Periurethral injection improves intrinsic sphincter function.
  - Newer minimally invasive techniques (eg, tension-free vaginal tape) address the distal defect.
• At least two thirds of surgically treated patients should have substantial improvement or cure.

CATHETER CARE
• Use **only** for chronic urinary retention, nonhealing pressure ulcers in incontinent patients, and when requested by patients or families to promote comfort.
• Use closed drainage system only; avoid topical or systemic antibiotics or catheters treated with antibiotics. Silver alloy hydrogel catheters reduce UTI by 27% to 73%.
• Bacteriuria is universal; treat only if symptoms (ie, fever, inanition, anorexia, delirium), or if bacteriuria persists after catheter removal.
• How to culture from catheter: through the port, not from the bag.
• Replace catheter if symptomatic bacteriuria occurs, then culture urine.
• Nursing facility patients with catheters should be kept in separate rooms.
• For acute retention catheterize for 7–10 d, then do voiding trial after catheter removal, never clamping.
• **Replacing Catheters:** Routine replacement not necessary. Changing every 4–6 wk is reasonable to prevent blockage. Patients with recurrent blockage need increased fluid intake and dilute acetic acid bladder irrigation.

VISUAL IMPAIRMENT

DEFINITION
Visual acuity 20/40 or worse; severe visual impairment (legal blindness) 20/200 or worse

EVALUATION
Acuity Testing
Near Vision: Check each eye independently with glasses using handheld Rosenbaum card at 14" or Lighthouse Near Acuity Test at 16".
Far Vision: Snellen wall chart at 20'
Visual Fields: By confrontation

Ophthalmoscopic Evaluation
Tonometry: Using Tono-pen (portable)

Causes of Visual Impairment in Decreasing Order of Frequency
Refractive Error: Most common cause of impairment
Cataracts: Lens opacity on ophthalmoscopic examination. Risk factors: Age, sun exposure, smoking, corticosteroids, diabetes mellitus.
Age-Related Macular Degeneration (ARMD): Atrophy of cells in the central macular region of retinal pigmented epithelium; on ophthalmoscopic examination white-yellow patches (drusen) or hemorrhage and scars in advanced stages. Risk factors: Age, sunlight exposure, family hx, white race.
Diabetic Retinopathy: Microaneurysms, dot and blot hemorrhages on ophthalmoscopy with proliferative retinopathy ischemia and vitreous hemorrhage. Risk factors: Chronic hyperglycemia.
Glaucoma: Intraocular pressure > 21 mm Hg, optic cupping and nerve head atrophy, and loss of peripheral visual fields. Risk factors: Black race, age, family hx, elevated eye pressures.

MANAGEMENT
Prevention
Biennial full eye examinations for persons > 65 years of age, annually for diabetic persons

Nonpharmacologic Interventions
ARMD: Photocoagulation for wet form: monitor using Amsler grid daily.
Cataract Surgery: AHCPR guidelines (AHCPR Publication No. 93-0542): if acuity 20/50 or worse with symptoms of poor functional acuity; or if 20/40 or better with disabling glare or frequent exposure to low light situations, diplopia, disparity between eyes, or occupational need; or when cataract removal will treat another lens-induced disease (eg, glaucoma); or when cataract coexists with retinal disease requiring unrestricted monitoring (eg, diabetic retinopathy)
Diabetic Retinopathy: Laser treatment of proliferative retinopathy or macular edema

Glaucoma Surgery: Open angle—laser trabeculoplasty or surgical trabeculectomy; angle closure—laser iridotomy; used primarily when pressures are poorly controlled by topical agents or when visual loss progresses

Pharmacologic Interventions

ARMD: Zinc oxide 80 mg, cupric oxide 2 mg, β-carotene 15 mg, vitamin C 500 mg, and vitamin E 400 IU taken in divided doses bid reduces risk of progression (eg, *Ocuvite PreserVision* 2 tabs po bid).

Diabetic Retinopathy: Glycemic and BP control (see p 55)

Glaucoma: Treat when pressures are > 25 mm Hg or with optic nerve damage or visual field loss (see **Table 80**). Instill drops, close eye for 3–5 min to reduce systemic absorption.

Table 80. Agents for Treating Glaucoma			
Drug	Strength	Dosage	Comments (Metabolism)
Adrenergic Agonists (bottles with purple caps)			
Apraclonidine (*Iopidine*)	0.5%, 1%	1–2 drops tid	Low BP, fatigue, drowsiness, dry mouth, dry nose (unknown)
Brimonidine (*Alphagan*)	0.2%	1 drop tid	Low BP, fatigue, drowsiness, dry mouth, dry nose (L)
(*Alphagan P*)	0.15%	1 drop tid	Benzalkonium-chloride free
Dipivefrin (*AKPro, Propine*)	0.1%	1 drop bid	HTN, headache, tachycardia, arrhythmia (eye, L)
Epinephrine (*Epifrin, Glaucon*)	0.1%–2%	1 drop qd–bid	HTN, headache, tachycardia, arrhythmia (L)
Epinephrine borate (*Epinal*)	0.25%–0.5%	1 drop bid	HTN, headache, tachycardia, arrhythmia (L)
β-Blockers (bottles with blue or yellow caps)			Class side effects: hypotension, bradycardia, HF, bronchospasm, anxiety, confusion, hallucination, diarrhea, nausea, cramps, lethargy, weakness, masking of hypoglycemia, impotence (L)
Betaxolol (*Betoptic, Betoptic-S*)	0.25%, 0.5%	1–2 drops bid	
Carteolol (*Ocupress*)	1%	1 drop bid	
Levobunolol (*AKBeta, Betagan*)	0.25%, 0.5%	1 drop bid	
Metipranolol (*OptiPranolol*)	0.3%	1 drop bid	
Timolol drops (*Betimol, Timoptic*)	0.25%, 0.5%	1 drop bid	
Timolol gel (*Timoptic–XE*)	0.25%, 0.5%	1 drop qd (in AM)	
Miotics, Direct-Acting (bottles with green caps)			
Pilocarpine gel (*Pilopine HS*)	4%	1/2" qhs	Systemic cholinergic effects (tissues, K)
(*Ocusert*)	20, 40 μg/h	Weekly	

(continues)

Table 80. Agents for Treating Glaucoma (cont.)			
Drug	**Strength**	**Dosage**	**Comments (Metabolism)**
Pilocarpine (*Adsorbocarpine, Akarpine, Isopto Carpine, Pilagan, Pilocar, Piloptic, Pilostat*)	0.25%–10%	1 drop qid	Systemic cholinergic effects are rare (K)
Miotics, Cholinesterase Inhibitors (bottles with green caps)			Class side effects: cholinomimetic
Demecarium (*Humorsol*)	0.125%, 0.25%	1–2 drops bid	effects (sweating, tremor, headache, salivation), confusion, high or low BP, bradycardia, bronchoconstriction, urinary frequency, cramps, diarrhea, nausea, deterioration of mental status in persons with AD
Echothiophate (*Phospholine*)	0.03%–0.25%	1 drop bid	
Isoflurophate (*Floropryl*)	0.025% oint	0.25" strip 8–72 h	
Physostigmine (*Eserine, Fisostin, Isopto Eserine*)	0.25% oint	1" tid	(L)
Carbonic Anhydrase Inhibitors (bottles with orange caps)			
Topical			Caution in renal failure (K)
√ Brinzolamide (*Azopt*)	1%	1 drop tid	
√ Dorzolamide (*Trusopt*)	2%	1 drop tid	
Oral			Class side effects: fatigue, weight loss,
Acetazolamide (eg, *Diamox*)	125–500 mg, 500 mg SR	250–500 mg bid–qid, 500 SR bid	paresthesias, depression, COPD exacerbation, cramps, diarrhea, renal failure, blood dyscrasias, hypokalemia, acidosis; not recommended in renal failure (K)
Dichlorphenamide (*Daranide*)	50 mg	25–50 mg qd–tid	
Methazolamide (eg, *Neptazane*)	25–50 mg	50–100 mg bid–tid	(L,K)
Prostaglandin Analogues			Class side effects: change in eye color and periorbital tissues, hyperemia, itching; expensive (K, L)
Bimatoprost (*Lumigan*)	0.03%	1 drop hs	(L,K,F)
Latanoprost (*Xalatan*)	0.005%	1 drop hs	(L)
Travoprost (*Travatan*)	0.004%	1 drop hs	(L)
Unoprostone (*Rescula*)	0.15%	1 drop hs	(L)
Other Topical			
Dorzolamide/timolol (*Cosopt*)	0.2%, 0.05%	1 drop bid	Unusual taste, ocular itching, burning (K, L)

Note: Patients may not know names of drugs but instead refer to them by the color of the bottle cap. The usual color scheme is referenced above. √ = preferred for treating older persons.

Low-Vision Rehabilitation and Aids

Refer patients with uncompensated visual loss causing functional deficits. Aids include optical, nonoptical, low- and high-technology devices. Strategies include improved illumination, increased contrast, magnification, and auditory and tactile feedback. Environmental modifications include using color contrast, floor lamps to reduce glare, motion sensors to turn on lights, high-technology options including video magnification with closed-circuit television and word processing programs to enlarge text.

Dry Eye Syndrome

Symptoms: Itchy or sandy (foreign body sensation)

Etiology: Many; consider autoimmune (Sjögren's syndrome), drug-induced, refer to ophthalmology for diagnostic assistance.

Therapy:
- Artificial tear formulations (eg, *HypoTears*)
- Viscoelastic tear formulations containing either chondroitin sulfate or hyaluronic acid are not better than artificial tears.
- Cyclosporine ophthalmic emulsion 0.05% (*Restasis*) 1 gtt OU q 12 h. Indicated when tear production is suppressed by inflammation. Does not increase tears in persons using topical anti-inflammatories or punctal plugs. Side effects: burning, hyperemia, discharge, pain, blurring.

Acute Conjunctivitis

Symptoms: Red eye, foreign body sensation, discharge, photophobia

Signs: Conjunctival hyperemia and discharge. Visual acuity, pupillary light reflexes, and visual fields are normal. If eye functions are abnormal, refer to ophthalmology for urgent diagnosis.

Differential diagnosis: Acute iritis, acute glaucoma, episcleritis, or scleritis.

Etiology: Viral, bacterial, chlamydial, chemical, foreign body

Viral versus bacterial: Viral—profuse tearing, minimal exudation, preauricular adenopathy common, monocytes in stained scrapings and exudates;

bacterial—moderate tearing, profuse exudation, preauricular adenopathy uncommon, bacteria and polymorphonuclear cells in stained scrapings and exudates;

both—minimal itching, generalized hyperemia, occasional sore throat and fever.

Treatment: Majority are viral; treat symptoms with artificial tears and cool compresses. If purulent discharge, suspect bacterial; start broad-spectrum topical antibiotics (see **Table 81**). If severe, obtain culture and Gram's stain, then start treatment. If signs and symptoms fail to improve in 24–48 h, refer to ophthalmologist. If vision decreased or severe pain, refer to ophthalmologist immediately.

Other: Frequent hand washing and use of separate towels to avoid spread

| Table 81. Treatment for Acute Bacterial Conjunctivitis* |||
Agent	Formulations**	Comment
Ciprofloxacin (*Ciloxan Ophthalmic*)	0.3% sol, 0.3% oint	Very broad spectrum, well tolerated, a 1st choice in severe cases, expensive
Erythromycin ophthalmic (*AK-Mycin, Ilotycin*)	5 mg/gm oint	Good if staphylococcal blepharitis is present
Norfloxacin (*Chibroxin*)	0.3% sol	Very broad spectrum, well tolerated, a 1st choice in severe cases, expensive
Ofloxacin (*Floxin, Ocuflox Ophthalmic*)	0.3% sol, 0.3% oint	Very broad spectrum, well tolerated, a 1st choice in severe cases, expensive
Sulfacetamide sodium (*Sodium Sulamyd*)	10%, 30% drops, 10% oint	Same coverage as trimethoprim and polymyxin
Tobramycin (*AKTob, Tobrex*)	3 mg/gm oint, 3 mg/mL sol	Well tolerated, but more corneal toxic
Trimethoprim and polymyxin (*Polytrim*)	1 mg/mL, 10,000 IU/mL sol	Well tolerated but some gaps in coverage

* Do not use steroid or steroid-antibiotic preparations in initial treatment.
** In mild cases solution is applied qid and gel or ointments bid for 5–7 d. In more severe cases solution is applied q 2–3 h, ointment qid; as the eye improves, solution is applied qid and ointment, bid.

PREVENTION (See also p 134)
- Annual breast and pelvic and perineal examination
- Annual mammography if life expectancy >4 yr
- Discuss HRT risks/benefits with patients on treatment
- One negative Pap smear after 65 yr if low risk (ie, single established sexual partner, good prior screening, no hx of abnormal Pap smear)
- Osteoporosis evaluation (see p 116)

COMMON DISORDERS
Vulvar Diseases
Non-neoplastic:
- Lichen sclerosus—Occurs commonly on vulva of middle-aged and older women; causes 1/3 of benign vulvar lesions, extends to perirectal areas (classic hourglass appearance); lesions are white to pink macules or papules, may coalesce; symptoms are none or itching, soreness, or dyspareunia. Must biopsy for diagnosis: Associated with squamous cell cancer in 4% to 5%. R_x: Clobetasol propionate 0.05% qd–bid for 8–12 wk; then taper gradually to zero. Long-term follow-up advised.
- Squamous hyperplasia—Raised white keratinized lesions difficult to distinguish from vulvar intraepithelial neoplasia (VIN); must biopsy to exclude malignancy. R_x: Betamethasone dipropionate 0.05% for 6–8 wk, then 1% hydrocortisone if symptoms persist; long-term follow-up advised.

Neoplastic:
- VIN—Most often seen in postmenopausal women; asymptomatic or may cause pruritus; appear as hypo- or hyperpigmented keratinized lesions; often multifocal; inspection ± colposcopy of the entire vulva with biopsy of most worrisome lesions; lesions graded on degree of atypia. R_x: surgical or other ablative therapy.
- Vulvar malignancy—Half of cases occur in women aged > 70 yr; 80% are squamous cell, with melanoma, sarcoma, basal cell, and adenocarcinoma < 20%; biopsy any suspicious lesion. R_x: radical surgery is preferred treatment.

Postmenopausal Bleeding
Bleeding after 1 yr of amenorrhea:
- Exclude malignancy, identify source, treat symptoms.
- Examine genitalia, perineum, rectum.
- If endometrial source, use endometrial biopsy or vaginal probe ultrasound to assess endometrial thickness (< 5 mm virtually excludes malignancy).
- D&C when endometrium not otherwise adequately assessed.
- Women on combination continuous estrogen and progesterone who bleed after 12 mo need evaluation.
- Those on cyclic replacement with bleeding at unexpected times (ie, bleeding other than during the second week of progesterone therapy) need evaluation.
- Women on unopposed estrogen who bleed at any time need evaluation.

Hot Flushes

- Vasomotor symptoms respond to estrogen (see **Table 83**) in dose-response fashion; start low dose, titrate to effect.
- If estrogen cannot be taken, try one of the less effective alternatives:
  - megestrol (*Megace*): [T: 20, 40] 20 mg qd-bid
  - venlafaxine 75 mg/d
  - paroxetine 20 mg/d
  - gabapentin (*Neurontin*) usually 300–600 tid [C: 100, 300, 400; T: 600, 800; S: 250/5 mL]
  - clonidine (*Catapres, Duraclon*): [T: 0.1, 0.2, 0.3] 0.1–0.3 mg/d; use lowest effective dose, watch for orthostatic ↓ BP and rebound ↑ BP if used intermittently

Vaginal Prolapse

- Child-bearing and other causes of increased intra-abdominal pressure weaken connective tissue and muscles supporting the genital organs, leading to prolapse.
- Symptoms include: Pelvic pressure, back pain, fecal or urinary incontinence, difficulty evacuating the rectum. Symptoms may be present even with mild prolapse.
- The degree of prolapse and organs involved dictate therapy; no therapy if asymptomatic.
- Estrogen and Kegel's exercises may help in mild cases.
- Pessary or surgery indicated with greater symptoms. Surgery needed for 4th-degree symptomatic prolapse.
- Precise anatomic defect(s) dictates the surgical approach.
- A common (ACOG) classification for degrees of prolapse:
  - First degree—extension to mid-vagina
  - Second degree—approaching hymenal ring
  - Third degree—at hymenal ring
  - Fourth degree—beyond hymenal ring

Atrophic Vaginitis (See p 156)

HORMONE THERAPY
Estrogen Therapy

- Current understanding of risks for women > 65 yr old on estrogen replacement are given in **Table 82**.
- If the patient has a uterus, estrogen should be combined with progesterone to reduce risk of endometrial cancer.
- Some women prefer unopposed estrogen and annual endometrial biopsy.
- Common regimens are given in **Table 83**.
- Older women can get hot flushes if estrogen is discontinued suddenly. Tapering (eg, qod for 1–2 mo and then q 3 d for a few months) is better tolerated.

Table 82. Hormone Therapy Risks and Benefits		
Outcome	Estrogen	Estrogen/Progesterone
MI	unknown	↑*
PE	unknown	↑
Stroke	unknown	↑
Breast cancer	unknown†	↑‡
Hip fracture	possibly ↓	↓
Colon cancer	unknown	↓
Endometrial cancer	↑	no change or ↓
Gallbladder disease	↑	↑
Urogenital disease§	↓	↓
Dementia	unknown	↑

* No increase in CHD mortality
† No increase at 5-year follow-up in Women's Health Initiative (WHI)
‡ No clear increase in breast cancer mortality in WHI
§ Dyspareunia, UTI, vaginal dryness, and possibly incontinence

Contraindications:
- Undiagnosed vaginal bleeding
- Thromboembolic disease
- Breast cancer
- Endometrial cancer greater than Stage 1
- Possibly gallbladder disease
- Coronary heart disease

Table 83. Common Regimens for Hormone Therapy				
Preparation	Starting Dosage (mg/d)	Cyclic Dosing	Continuous Dosing	Formulations
Conjugated equine estrogen (*Premarin*)*	0.3–0.625	—	Daily	T: 0.3, 0.625, 0.9, 1.25, 2.5
Conjugated synthetic estrogen (*Cenestin*)	0.625	—	Daily	T: 0.625, 0.9, 1.25
Esterified estrogen (eg, *Estratab, Menest*)*	0.3–0.625	—	Daily	T: 0.3, 0.625, 1.25, 2.5
Estropipate (*Ogen, Ortho-Est*)*	0.625	—	Daily	T: 0.625, 1.25, 2.5
Micronized 17-β estradiol (*Estrace*)*	0.5–1	—	Daily	T: 0.5, 1, 2
Transdermal estrogen				
(*Alura*)	0.05–0.75	—	Biweekly	0.05 0.075, 0.1
(*Estraderm*)*	0.05–0.75	—	Biweekly	0.05, 0.1
(*Vivelle*)*	0.0375–0.05	—	Biweekly	0.025, 0.0375, 0.05, 0.075, 0.1
(*Climara*)*	0.025–0.05	—	Weekly	0.025, 0.05, 0.075, 0.1
(*FemPatch*)	0.025–0.05	—	Weekly	0.025

(*continues*)

Table 83. Common Regimens for Hormone Therapy (cont.)				
Preparation	Starting Dosage (mg/d)	Cyclic Dosing	Continuous Dosing	Formulations
Estradiol *and* norethindrone (*CombiPatch*)	0.05/0.14	Biweekly for 3 wk, 1wk off	—	0.05/0.14, 0.05/0.25
Medroxyprogesterone (*Cycrin, Provera*)	2.5–10	5–10 mg, days 1–14	2.5–5 mg daily	T: 2.5, 5, 10
Combinations				
Conjugated estrogen *and* medroxyprogesterone (*Prempro*)	0.625 0.45 1.5, 2.5, 5	—	Daily	Fixed dose 0.625/2.5 or 0.625/5 or 0.45/1.5
Conjugated estrogen *and* medroxyprogesterone (*Premphase*)	0.625 5	Days 1–28 Days 15–28	—	Fixed dose 0.625 days 1–14, 0.625/5 days 15–28
Estradiol *and* norethindrone (*FEMHRT 1/5*)	1 5	—	Daily	Fixed dose 1.0/5

* FDA approved for long-term use to prevent osteoporosis.

ASSESSMENT INSTRUMENTS

MINI-COG ASSESSMENT INSTRUMENT FOR DEMENTIA

The Mini-Cog assessment instrument combines an uncued 3-item recall test with a clock-drawing test (CDT). The Mini-Cog can be administered in about 3 minutes, requires no special equipment, and is relatively uninfluenced by level of education or language variations.

Administration
The test is administered as follows:

1. Instruct the patient to listen carefully to and remember 3 unrelated words and then to repeat the words.
2. Instruct the patient to draw the face of a clock, either on a blank sheet of paper, or on a sheet with the clock circle already drawn on the page. After the patient puts the numbers on the clock face, ask him or her to draw the hands of the clock to read a specific time, such as 11:20. These instructions can be repeated, but no additional instructions should be given. Give the patient as much time as needed to complete the task. The CDT serves as the recall distractor.
3. Ask the patient to repeat the 3 previously presented words.

Scoring
Give 1 point for each recalled word after the CDT distractor. Score 1–3.
  - A score of 0 indicates positive screen for dementia.
  - A score of 1 or 2 with an abnormal CDT indicates positive screen for dementia.
  - A score of 1 or 2 with a normal CDT indicates negative screen for dementia.
  - A score of 3 indicates negative screen for dementia.
The CDT is considered normal if all numbers are present in the correct sequence and position, and the hands readably display the requested time.

Source: Adapted in part from Borson S, Scanlan J, Brush M, Vitaliano P, Dokmak A. The mini-cog: a cognitive "vital signs" measure for dementia screening in multi-lingual elderly. *Int J Geriatr Psychiatry* 2000; 15(11):1021–1027.

PHYSICAL SELF-MAINTENANCE SCALE
(ACTIVITIES OF DAILY LIVING, OR ADLs)

In each category, circle the item that most closely describes the person's highest level of functioning and record the score assigned to that level (either 1 or 0) in the blank at the beginning of the category.

A. Toilet _____
1. Care for self at toilet completely; no incontinence 1
2. Needs to be reminded, or needs help in cleaning self, or has rare
   (weekly at most) accidents 0
3. Soiling or wetting while asleep more than once a week 0
4. Soiling or wetting while awake more than once a week 0
5. No control of bowels or bladder 0

B. Feeding _____
1. Eats without assistance 1
2. Eats with minor assistance at meal times and/or with special
   preparation of food, or help in cleaning up after meals 0
3. Feeds self with moderate assistance and is untidy 0
4. Requires extensive assistance for all meals 0
5. Does not feed self at all and resists efforts of others to feed him or her 0

C. Dressing _____
1. Dresses, undresses, and selects clothes from own wardrobe 1
2. Dresses and undresses self, with minor assistance 0
3. Needs moderate assistance in dressing and selection of clothes. 0
4. Needs major assistance in dressing, but cooperates with efforts of
   others to help 0
5. Completely unable to dress self and resists efforts of others to help 0

D. Grooming (neatness, hair, nails, hands, face, clothing) _____
1. Always neatly dressed, well-groomed, without assistance 1
2. Grooms self adequately with occasional minor assistance, eg, with shaving 0
3. Needs moderate and regular assistance or supervision with grooming 0
4. Needs total grooming care, but can remain well-groomed after help from others 0
5. Actively negates all efforts of others to maintain grooming 0

E. Physical Ambulation _____
1. Goes about grounds or city 1
2. Ambulates within residence on or about one block distant 0
3. Ambulates with assistance of (check one)
   a ( ) another person, b ( ) railing, c ( ) cane, d ( ) walker, e ( ) wheelchair 0
   1.____Gets in and out without help. 2.____Needs help getting in and out
4. Sits unsupported in chair or wheelchair, but cannot propel self without help 0
5. Bedridden more than half the time 0

F. Bathing _____
1. Bathes self (tub, shower, sponge bath) without help. 1
2. Bathes self with help getting in and out of tub. 0
3. Washes face and hands only, but cannot bathe rest of body 0
4. Does not wash self, but is cooperative with those who bathe him or her. 0
5. Does not try to wash self and resists efforts to keep him or her clean. 0

For scoring interpretation and source, see note following the next instrument.

INSTRUMENTAL ACTIVITIES OF DAILY LIVING SCALE (IADLs)

In each category, circle the item that most closely describes the person's highest level
of functioning and record the score assigned to that level (either 1 or 0) in the blank at
the beginning of the category.

A. Ability to Use Telephone _____
1. Operates telephone on own initiative; looks up and dials numbers. 1
2. Dials a few well-known numbers. 1
3. Answers telephone, but does not dial. 1
4. Does not use telephone at all. 0

B. Shopping _____
1. Takes care of all shopping needs independently. 1
2. Shops independently for small purchases. 1
3. Needs to be accompanied on any shopping trip. 0
4. Completely unable to shop. 0

C. Food Preparation _____

  1. Plans, prepares, and serves adequate meals independently. 1

  2. Prepares adequate meals if supplied with ingredients. 0

  3. Heats and serves prepared meals or prepares meals, but does not
   maintain adequate diet. 0

  4. Needs to have meals prepared and served. 0

D. Housekeeping

  1. Maintains house alone or with occasional assistance (eg, heavy-
   work domestic help). 1

  2. Performs light daily tasks such as dishwashing, bedmaking. 1

  3. Performs light daily tasks, but cannot maintain acceptable level of
   cleanliness. 1

  4. Needs help with all home maintenance tasks. 1

  5. Does not participate in any housekeeping tasks. 0

E. Laundry _____

  1. Does personal laundry completely. 1

  2. Launders small items; rinses socks, stockings, etc. 1

  3. All laundry must be done by others. 0

F. Mode of Transportation _____

  1. Travels independently on public transportation or drives own car. 1

  2. Arranges own travel via taxi, but does not otherwise use public
   transportation. 1

  3. Travels on public transportation when assisted or accompanied
   by another. 1

  4. Travel limited to taxi or automobile with assistance of another. 0

  5. Does not travel at all. 0

G. Responsibility for Own Medications _____

  1. Is responsible for taking medication in correct dosages at correct time. 1

  2. Takes responsibility if medication is prepared in advance in separate
   dosages. 0

  3. Is not capable of dispensing own medication. 0

H. Ability to Handle Finances _____

  1. Manages financial matters independently (budgets, writes checks,
   pays rent and bills, goes to bank); collects and keeps track of income. 1

  2. Manages day-to-day purchases, but needs help with banking,
   major purchases, etc. 1

  3. Incapable of handling money. 0

Scoring Interpretation: For ADLs, the total score ranges from 0 to 6, and for IADLs, from 0 to 8. In some categories, only the highest level of function receives a 1; in others, two or more levels have scores of 1 because each describes competence that represents some minimal level of function. These screens are useful for indicating specifically how a person is performing at the present time. When they are also used over time, they serve as documentation of a person's functional improvement or deterioration.

Source: Lawton MP, Brody EM. Assessment of older people: self-maintaining and instrumental activities of daily living. *Gerontologist* 1969, 9:179–186. Copyright by the Gerontological Society of America. Reproduced by permission of the publisher.

GERIATRIC DEPRESSION SCALE (GDS, SHORT FORM)

Choose the best answer for how you felt over the past week.

  1. Are you basically satisfied with your life?   yes/**no**

  2. Have you dropped many of your activities and interests?   **yes**/no

  3. Do you feel that your life is empty?   **yes**/no

  4. Do you often get bored?   **yes**/no

5. Are you in good spirits most of the time?	yes/**no**
6. Are you afraid that something bad is going to happen to you?	**yes**/no
7. Do you feel happy most of the time?	yes/**no**
8. Do you often feel helpless?	**yes**/no
9. Do you prefer to stay at home, rather than going out and doing new things?	**yes**/no
10. Do you feel you have more problems with memory than most?	**yes**/no
11. Do you think it is wonderful to be alive now?	yes/**no**
12. Do you feel pretty worthless the way you are now?	**yes**/no
13. Do you feel full of energy?	yes/**no**
14. Do you feel that your situation is hopeless?	**yes**/no
15. Do you think that most people are better off than you are?	**yes**/no

Score 1 point for each bolded answer. Cut-off: normal (0–5), above 5 suggests depression.

Source: Courtesy of Jerome A. Yesavage, MD. For 30 translations of the GDS, see
www.stanford.edu/~yesavage/GDS.html
For additional information on administration and scoring, refer to the following references:
1. Sheikh JI, Yesavage JA. Geriatric Depression Scale: recent evidence and development of a shorter version. *Clin Gerontol.*
1986;5:165–172.
2. Feher EP, Larrabee GJ, Crook TH 3rd. Factors attenuating the validity of the Geriatric Depression Scale in a dementia
population. *J Am Geriatr Soc.* 1992;40:906–909.
3. Yesavage JA, Brink TL, Rose TL, et al. Development and validation of a geriatric depression rating scale: a preliminary
report. *J Psychiatr Res.* 1983;17:27.

BRIEF HEARING LOSS SCREENER

	Points
1. Age:_____	_____
If age > 70 years = 1 point	
2. Sex: Male_____ Female_____	_____
If male = 1 point	
3. Highest grade attended:	_____
12th grade or less _____	
higher than 12th grade_____	
If ≤ 12th grade = 1 point	
4. Have you ever had deafness or trouble hearing with one or both ears?	0
Yes_____, continue to Question #5.	
No_____, go to Question #6.	
No points assigned to this question.	
5. Did you ever see a doctor about it?	_____
Yes_____No_____	
If "Yes" = 2 points	
6. Without a hearing aid, can you usually hear and understand what a person says without seeing his/her face if that person whispers to you from across the room?	_____
Yes_____No_____	
If "No" = 1 point	
7. Without a hearing aid, can you usually hear and understand what a person says without seeing his/her face if that person talks to you in a normal voice from across the room?	_____
Yes_____No_____	
If "No" = 2 points	
TOTAL	_____

3 or more points is a positive score indicating the need for further evaluation.

Test Characteristics of This Screener With Established Hearing Loss Criteria

	Sensitivity	Specificity	Pos Predictive Value	Neg Predictive Value
Ventry-Weinstein criteria	80%	80%	45%	95%
High-frequency pure-tone average	59%	88%	76%	77%

Source: Reuben DB, Walsh K, Moore AA, et al. Hearing loss in community-dwelling older persons: national prevalence data and identification using simple questions. *J Am Geriatr Soc.* 1998;46:1011. Reprinted with permission.

PERFORMANCE-ORIENTED MOBILITY ASSESSMENT (POMA)

Balance

Chair: Instructions: Place a hard armless chair against a wall. The following maneuvers are tested.

1. Sitting down
   - 0 = unable without help or collapses (plops) into chair *or* lands off center of chair
   - 1 = able and does not meet criteria for 0 or 2
   - 2 = sits in a smooth, safe motion *and* ends with buttocks against back of chair and thighs centered on chair
2. Sitting balance
   - 0 = unable to maintain position (marked slide forward or leans forward or to side)
   - 1 = eans in chair slightly or slight increased distance from buttocks to back of chair
   - 2 = steady, safe, upright.
3. Arising
   - 0 = unable without help or loses balance or requires > three attempts
   - 1 = able but requires three attempts
   - 2 = able in ≤ two attempts
4. Immediate standing balance (first 5 seconds)
   - 0 = unsteady, marked staggering, moves feet, marked trunk sway or grabs object for support
   - 1 = steady but uses walker or cane or mild staggering but catches self without grabbing object
   - 2 = steady without walker or cane or other support

Stand

5a. Side-by-side standing balance
   - 0 = unable *or* unsteady *or* holds ≤ 3 seconds
   - 1 = able *but* uses cane, walker, or other support *or* holds for 4–9 seconds
   - 2 = narrow stance without support for 10 seconds

5b. Timing ___.__ seconds

6. Pull test (person at maximum position attained in #5, examiner stands behind and exerts mild pull back at waist)
   - 0 = begins to fall
   - 1 = takes more than two steps back
   - 2 = fewer than two steps backward and steady

7a. Able to stand on right leg unsupported
   - 0 = unable *or* holds onto any objects *or* able for < 3 seconds
   - 1 = able for 3 or 4 seconds
   - 2 = able for 5 seconds

7b. Timing ___.__ seconds

8a. Able to stand on left leg unsupported
- 0 = unable *or* holds onto any object *or* able for < 3 seconds
- 1 = able for 3 or 4 seconds
- 2 = able for 5 seconds

8b. Timing ___ . __ seconds

9a. Semitandem stand
- 0 = unable to stand with one foot half in front of other with feet touching *or* begins to fall *or* holds for ≤ 3 seconds
- 1 = able for 4 to 9 seconds
- 2 = able to semitandem stand for 10 seconds

9b. Timing ___ . __ seconds

10a. Tandem stand
- 0 = unable to stand with one foot in front of other *or* begins to fall *or* holds for ≤ 3 seconds
- 1 = able for 4 to 9 seconds
- 2 = able to tandem stand for 10 seconds

10b. Timing ___ . __ seconds

11. Bending over (to pick up a pen off floor)
- 0 = unable *or* is unsteady
- 1 = able, but requires more than one attempt to get up
- 2 = able and is steady

12. Toe stand
- 0 = unable
- 1 = able but < 3 seconds
- 2 = able for 3 seconds

13. Heel stand
- 0 = unable
- 1 = able but < 3 seconds
- 2 = able for 3 seconds

Gait: Instructions: Person stands with examiner, walks down 10-ft walkway (measured). Ask the person to walk down walkway, turn, and walk back. The person should use customary walking aid.

Bare Floor (flat, even surface)
1. Type of surface: 1 = linoleum or tile; 2 = wood; 3 = cement or concrete; 4 = other _____ [not included in scoring]
2. Initiation of gait (immediately after told to "go")
   - 0 = any hesitancy or multiple attempts to start
   - 1 = no hesitancy
3. Path (estimated in relation to tape measure). Observe excursion of foot closest to tape measure over middle 8 feet of course.
   - 0 = marked deviation
   - 1 = mild or moderate deviation *or* uses walking aid
   - 2 = straight without walking aid
4. Missed step (trip or loss of balance)
   - 0 = yes, and would have fallen *or* more than two missed steps
   - 1 = yes, but appropriate attempt to recover *and* no more than two missed steps
   - 2 = none
5. Turning (while walking)
   - 0 = almost falls
   - 1 = mild staggering, but catches self, uses walker or cane
   - 2 = steady, without walking aid
6. Step over obstacles (to be assessed in a separate walk with two shoes placed on course 4 feet apart)
   - 0 = begins to fall at any obstacle *or* unable *or* walks around any obstacle *or* > two missed steps

1 = able to step over all obstacles, but some staggering and catches self *or* one
    to two missed steps
2 = able and steady at stepping over all four obstacles with no missed steps

Source: Courtesy of Mary E. Tinetti, MD. Adapted with permission.

ABNORMAL INVOLUNTARY MOVEMENT SCALE (AIMS)

Examination Procedure
Either before or after completing the examination procedure, observe the patient
unobtrusively, at rest (eg, in waiting room). The chair to be used in this examination
should be a hard, firm one without arms.

1. Ask patient to remove shoes and socks.
2. Ask patient whether there is anything in his/her mouth (ie, gum, candy, etc) and if
   there is, to remove it.
3. Ask patient about the **current** condition of his/her teeth. Ask patient if he/she wears
   dentures. Do teeth or dentures bother patient **now**?
4. Ask patient whether he/she notices any movements in mouth, face, hands, or feet. If
   yes, ask to describe and to what extent they **currently** bother patient or interfere
   with his/her activities.
5. Have patient sit in chair with hands on knees, legs slightly apart, and feet flat on
   floor. (Look at entire body for movements while in this position.)
6. Ask patient to sit with hands hanging unsupported. If male, between legs, if female
   and wearing a dress, hanging over knees. (Observe hands and other body areas.)
7. Ask patient to open mouth. (Observe tongue at rest within mouth.) Do this twice.
8. Ask patient to protrude tongue. (Observe abnormalities of tongue movement.) Do this
   twice.
9. Ask patient to tap thumb with each finger as rapidly as possible for 10–15 seconds;
   separately with right hand, then with left hand. (Observe facial and leg movements.)
10. Flex and extend patient's left and right arms (one at a time). (Note any rigidity.)
11. Ask patient to stand up. (Observe in profile. Observe all body areas again, hips
    included.)
12. Ask patient to extend both arms outstretched in front with palms down. (Observe
    trunk, legs, and mouth.)
13. Have patient walk a few paces, turn, and walk back to chair. (Observe hands and
    gait.) Do this twice.

Instructions: Complete examination procedure before making ratings. Rate highest
severity observed.
Code:
    1 None
    2 Minimal, may be extreme normal
    3 Mild
    4 Moderate
    5 Severe

Facial and Oral Movements

1. Muscles of facial expression (eg, movements of forehead, eyebrows, periorbital area, cheeks; including frowning, blinking, smiling, grimacing)

    1   2   3   4   5

2. Lips and perioral area (eg, puckering, pouting, smacking)

    1   2   3   4   5

3. Jaw (eg, biting, clenching, chewing, mouth opening, lateral movement)

    1   2   3   4   5

4. Tongue (rate only increase in movement both in and out of mouth, NOT inability to sustain movement)

    1   2   3   4   5

Extremity Movements

5. Upper (arms, wrists, hands, fingers). Include choreic movements (ie, rapid, objectively purposeless, irregular, spontaneous), athetoid movements (ie, slow, irregular, complex, serpentine). Do NOT include tremor (ie, repetitive, regular, rhythmic).

    1   2   3   4   5

6. Lower (legs, knees, ankles, toes). (Eg, lateral knee movement, foot tapping, heel dropping, foot squirming, inversion and eversion of foot)

    1   2   3   4   5

Trunk Movements

7. Neck, shoulders, hips (eg, rocking, twisting, squirming, pelvic gyrations)

    1   2   3   4   5

Global Judgments

8. Severity of abnormal movements
    1 None, normal
    2 Minimal
    3 Mild
    4 Moderate
    5 Severe

9. Incapacitation due to abnormal movements
    1 None, normal
    2 Minimal
    3 Mild
    4 Moderate
    5 Severe

10. Patient's awareness of abnormal movements (rate only patient's report)
    1 No awareness
    2 Aware, no distress
    3 Aware, mild distress
    4 Aware, moderate distress
    5 Aware, severe distress

Dental Status

11. Current problems with teeth and/or dentures

    1 No

    2 Yes

12. Does patient usually wear dentures?

    1 No

    2 Yes

Source: Adapted from Department of Health and Human Services, Public Health Service, Alcohol, Drug Abuse and Mental Health Administration, National Institute of Mental Health. *Treatment Strategies in Schizophrenia Study.* ADM-117. Revised 1985.

PAIN SCALES FOR ASSESSING PAIN INTENSITY

Use copies of pain scales that are large enough for older patients to see comfortably (14-point font or larger).

Faces Pain Scale

Place an X under the face that best represents the severity or intensity of your pain right now.

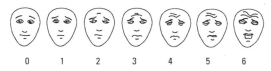

Source: Reprinted from *Pain*, 41(2), Bien D, Reeve R, Champion G, et al. The Faces Pain Scale for the self-assessment of the severity of pain experienced by children: development and initial validation, and preliminary investigation for ratio scale properties. 139–150, Copyright 1990, with permission from the International Society for the Study of Pain.

0–10 Numeric Rating Scales

Verbal: On a scale of 0–10, with 0 being no pain and 10 being the most intense pain imaginable, what would you rate the severity or intensity of your pain right now? _____

Source: Keela Herr, 2004.

Visual: Circle the number that best represents the severity or intensity of your pain right now.

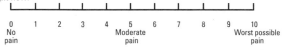

Source: Carr DB, Jacox AK, Chapman CR, et al. *Acute Pain Management: Operative Medical Procedures and Trauma.* Clinical Practice Guideline No. 1. Rockville, MD: AHCPR, Public Health Service, US Dept of Health and Human Services; February 1992. AHCPR Publication No. 92-0032.

Verbal Descriptor Scale

Place an X beside the words that best describe the severity or intensity of your pain right now. Mark one set of words.

———The Most Intense Pain Imaginable
———Very Severe Pain
———Severe Pain
———Moderate Pain
———Mild Pain
———Slight Pain
———No Pain

Source: Keela Herr, 2004.

Reference

AGS Panel on Persistent Pain in Older Persons. The management of persistent pain in older persons. *J Am Geriatr Soc.* 2002; 50(6, Suppl): S205–S224.

STUDY ID #: _____   HOSPITAL #: _____

DO NOT WRITE ABOVE THIS LINE

Brief Pain Inventory (Short Form)

Date: ___ / ___ / ___   Time: _____

Name: _____

Last   First   Middle Initial

1. Throughout our lives, most of us have had pain from time to time (such as minor headaches, sprains, and toothaches). Have you had pain other than these every-day kinds of pain today?

1. Yes   2. No

2. On the diagram, shade in the areas where you feel pain. Put an X on the area that hurts the most.

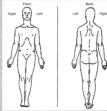

3. Please rate your pain by circling the one number that best describes your pain at its worst in the last 24 hours.

0   1   2   3   4   5   6   7   8   9   10
No   Pain as bad as
Pain   you can imagine

4. Please rate your pain by circling the one number that best describes your pain at its least in the last 24 hours.

0   1   2   3   4   5   6   7   8   9   10
No   Pain as bad as
Pain   you can imagine

5. Please rate your pain by circling the one number that best describes your pain on the average.

0   1   2   3   4   5   6   7   8   9   10
No   Pain as bad as
Pain   you can imagine

6. Please rate your pain by circling the one number that tells how much pain you have right now.

0   1   2   3   4   5   6   7   8   9   10
No   Pain as bad as
Pain   you can imagine

Page 1 of 2

Date: ___/___/___			Time: _____
Name:			
	Last	First	Middle Initial

7. What treatments or medications are you receiving for your pain?

_____

8. In the last 24 hours, how much relief have pain treatments or medications provided? Please circle the one percentage that most shows how much relief you have received.

| 0% | 10% | 20% | 30% | 40% | 50% | 60% | 70% | 80% | 90% | 100% |
| No Relief | | | | | | | | | | Complete Relief |

9. Circle the one number that describes how, during the past 24 hours, pain has interfered with your:

A. General Activity

| 0 | 1 | 2 | 3 | 4 | 5 | 6 | 7 | 8 | 9 | 10 |
| Does not Interfere | | | | | | | | | | Completely Interferes |

B. Mood

| 0 | 1 | 2 | 3 | 4 | 5 | 6 | 7 | 8 | 9 | 10 |
| Does not Interfere | | | | | | | | | | Completely Interferes |

C. Walking Ability

| 0 | 1 | 2 | 3 | 4 | 5 | 6 | 7 | 8 | 9 | 10 |
| Does not Interfere | | | | | | | | | | Completely Interferes |

D. Normal Work (includes both work outside the home and housework)

| 0 | 1 | 2 | 3 | 4 | 5 | 6 | 7 | 8 | 9 | 10 |
| Does not Interfere | | | | | | | | | | Completely Interferes |

E. Relations with other people

| 0 | 1 | 2 | 3 | 4 | 5 | 6 | 7 | 8 | 9 | 10 |
| Does not Interfere | | | | | | | | | | Completely Interferes |

F. Sleep

| 0 | 1 | 2 | 3 | 4 | 5 | 6 | 7 | 8 | 9 | 10 |
| Does not Interfere | | | | | | | | | | Completely Interferes |

G. Enjoyment of life

| 0 | 1 | 2 | 3 | 4 | 5 | 6 | 7 | 8 | 9 | 10 |
| Does not Interfere | | | | | | | | | | Completely Interferes |

Worst pain, or the arithmetic mean of the 4 severity items (items 3, 4, 5, and 6), can be used as measures of pain severity. The arithmetic mean of the 7 interference item (items 9A-G) can be used as a measure of pain interference. Scores on the BPI pain severity items are defined as mild (1–4), moderate (5–6), and severe (7–10). The tool can be used to follow the course of pain and response to interventions.

AUA SYMPTOM INDEX FOR BPH

Questions to be answered (circle one number on each line)	Not at all	Less than 1 time in 5	Less than half the time	About half the time	More than half the time	Almost always
1. Over the past month or so, how often have you had a sensation of not emptying your bladder completely after you finished urinating?	0	1	2	3	4	5
2. Over the past month or so, how often have you had to urinate again less than two hours after you finished urinating?	0	1	2	3	4	5
3. Over the past month or so, how often have you found you stopped and started again several times when you urinated?	0	1	2	3	4	5
4. Over the past month or so, how often have you found it difficult to postpone urination?	0	1	2	3	4	5
5. Over the past month or so, how often have you had a weak urinary stream?	0	1	2	3	4	5
6. Over the past month or so, how often have you had to push or strain to begin urination?	0	1	2	3	4	5
7. Over the last month, how many times did you most typically get up to urinate from the time you went to bed at night until the time you got up in the morning?	(none) 0	(1 time) 1	(2 times) 2	(3 times) 3	(4 times) 4	(5 or more times) 5

AUA Symptom Score = sum of questions 1–7 = _____. For interpretation, see p 144.

Source: Barry MJ, Fowler FJ Jr, O'Leary MP et al. The American Urological Association symptom index for benign prostatic hyperplasia. *J Urol.* 1992;148(5):1549–1557. Reprinted with permission.

MEDICATION APPROPRIATENESS ASSESSMENT

To assess the appropriateness of a drug, the following questions should be considered in view of the patient's medical problems and current medications. For combination drugs, the questions should be considered for each drug. See also p 9.

- Is there an indication for the drug?
- Is the medication effective for the condition?
- Is the dosage correct?
- Are the directions correct?
- Are the directions practical?

- Are there clinically significant drug-drug interactions?
- Are there clinically significant drug-disease/condition interactions?
- Is there unnecessary duplication with other drug(s)?
- Is the duration of therapy acceptable?
- Is this drug the least expensive alternative compared with others of equal utility?

Source: Adapted from Hanlon JT, Schmader KE, Samsa GP, et al. A method for assessing drug therapy appropriateness. *J Clin Epidemiol* 1992; 45(10):1045–51, copyright (1992) with permission from Elsevier.

US Health Care Financing Administration (in 2001 renamed Centers for Medicare and Medicaid Services, or CMS) regulations regarding the use of certain medications in nursing homes are contained in the Omnibus Budget Reconciliation Act (OBRA) of 1987.

ANTIDEPRESSANT MEDICATIONS

Table 84. Recommended Maximum Doses of Antidepressants		
Drug	Usual Max Daily Dose (mg) for Age ≥ 65	Usual Max Daily Dose (mg)
Amitriptyline (*Elavil*)	150	300
Amoxapine (*Asendin*)	200	400
Desipramine (*Norpramin*)	150	300
Doxepin (*Adapin, Sinequan*)	150	300
Imipramine (*Tofranil*)	150	300
Maprotiline (*Ludiomil*)	150	300
Nortriptyline (*Aventyl, Pamelor*)	75	150
Protriptyline (*Vivactil*)	30	60
Trazodone (*Desyrel*)	300	600
Trimipramine (*Surmontil*)	150	300

ANTIPSYCHOTIC MEDICATIONS

Indications for appropriate use of antipsychotic medications are outlined in OBRA. In addition to psychotic disorders, these indications include specific nonpsychotic behavior associated with organic mental syndromes:

- Agitated psychotic symptoms (biting, kicking, scratching, assertive and belligerent behavior, sexual aggressiveness) that present a danger to themselves or others or interfere with family's and/or staff's ability to provide care (activities of daily living, or ADLs)
- Psychotic symptoms (hallucinations, delusions, paranoia)
- Continuous (24-h) crying out and screaming

Behavior less responsive to antipsychotic therapy includes:

- Repetitive, bothersome behavior (ie, pacing, wandering, repeated statements or words, calling out, fidgeting)
- Poor self-care
- Unsociability
- Indifference to surroundings
- Uncooperative behavior
- Restlessness
- Impaired memory
- Anxiety
- Depression
- Insomnia

If antipsychotic therapy is to be used for one or more of these symptoms only, then the use of antipsychotic agents is inappropriate. Because of their anticholinergic properties, antipsychotic agents may worsen these symptoms, especially symptoms of sedation and lethargy, as well as enhance "confusion."

Selection of an antipsychotic agent should be based on the side-effect profile since all antipsychotic agents are equally effective at equivalent doses. Coadministration of two or more antipsychotics does not have any pharmacologic basis or clinical advantage. Coadministration of two or more antipsychotic agents does not improve clinical response and increases the potential for side effects.

Once behavior control is obtained, assess patient to determine if precipitating event (stress from drugs, fluid or electrolyte changes, infection, changes in environment) has been resolved or patient has accommodated to the environment or situation. Determine whether the antipsychotic can be decreased in dose or tapered off completely by monitoring selected target symptoms for which the antipsychotic therapy was initiated. OBRA 1987 requires attempts at dose reduction within a 6-month period unless documented as to why this cannot be done. Identifying target symptoms is essential for adequate monitoring. Because of side effects, intermittent use (not prn) is preferable (ie, only when patient has behavior warranting use of these agents). For the recommended doses of antipsychotics, see **Table 85**.

Table 85. Recommended Maximum Doses of Antipsychotics			
Drug	Usual Max Daily Dose (mg) for Age ≥ 65	Usual Max Daily Dose (mg)	Daily Oral Dose (mg) for Residents with Organic Mental Syndromes
Acetophenazine (*Tindal*)	150	300	20
Chlorpromazine (*Thorazine*)	800	1600	75
Chlorprothixene (*Taractan*)	800	1600	75
Clozapine (*Clozaril*)	25	450	50
Fluphenazine (*Prolixin*)	20	40	4
Haloperidol (*Haldol*)	50	100	4
Loxapine (*Loxitane*)	125	250	10
Mesoridazine (*Serentil*)	250	500	25
Molindone (*Moban*)	112	225	10
Olanzapine (*Zyprexa*)	—	20	10
Quetiapine (*Seroquel*)	—	800	200
Perphenazine (*Trilafon*)	32	64	8
Promazine (*Sparine*)	50	500	150
Risperidone (*Risperdal*)	1	16	2
Thioridazine (*Mellaril*)	400	800	75
Thiothixene (*Navane*)	30	60	7
Trifluoperazine (*Stelazine*)	40	80	8
Trifluopromazine (*Vesprin*)	100	20	—

ANXIOLYTIC MEDICATIONS
The use of anxiolytics is acceptable as long as other disease processes that could explain anxious behavior have been excluded. Daily use, at any dose, is for less than 4 continuous months, unless an attempt at dose reduction is unsuccessful. Proper indications include:
• Generalized anxiety disorder
• Organic mental syndrome (including dementia associated with agitation)
• Panic disorders
• Anxiety associated with other psychiatric disorder (eg, depression, adjustment disorder)

Table 86. Recommended Maximum Doses of Anxiolytics*		
Drug	Usual Daily Dose (mg) for Age ≥ 65	Usual Daily Dose (mg) for Age < 65
Alprazolam (Xanax)	2	4
Clorazepate (Tranxene)	30	60
Chlordiazepoxide (Librium)	40	100
Diazepam (Valium)	20	60
Halazepam (Paxipam)	80	160
Lorazepam (Ativan)	3	6
Meprobamate (Miltown)	600	1600
Oxazepam (Serax)	60	90
Prazepam (Centrax)	30	60

*CMS-OBRA guidelines strongly urge clinicians not to use barbiturates, glutethimide, and ethchlorvynol because of their side effects, pharmacokinetics, and addiction potential in the elderly person. Also, CMS discourages use of long-acting benzodiazepines in treating the elderly person.

HYPNOTIC MEDICATIONS

Hypnotics are allowed for 10 continuous days of use. If three unsuccessful attempts at dose reduction occur, then it is clinically contraindicated to reduce.

Table 87. Recommended Maximum Doses of Hypnotics*		
Drug	Usual Max Single Dose (mg) for Age ≥ 65	Usual Max Single Dose (mg)
Alprazolam (Xanax)	0.25	1.5
Amobarbital (Amytal)	150	300
Butabarbital (Butisol)	100	200
Chloral hydrate (Noctec)	750	1500
Chloral hydrate (various)	500	1000
Diphenhydramine (Benadryl)	25	50
Ethchlorvynol (Placidyl)	500	1000
Flurazepam (Dalmane)	15	30
Glutethimide (Doriden)	500	1000
Halazepam (Paxipam)	20	40
Hydroxyzine (Atarax)	50	100
Lorazepam (Ativan)	1	2
Methyprylon (Noludar)	200	400
Oxazepam (Serax)	15	30
Phenobarbital (Nembutal)	100	200
Secobarbital (Seconal)	100	200
Temazepam (Restoril)	15	30
Triazolam (Halcion)	0.125	0.5

*CMS-OBRA guidelines strongly urge clinicians not to use barbiturates, glutethimide, and ethchlorvynol because of their side effects, pharmacokinetics, and addiction potential in the elderly person. Also, CMS discourages use of long-acting benzodiazepines in treating the elderly person.

CMS CRITERIA: INAPPROPRIATE DRUG USE IN NURSING HOMES

On July 1, 1999, HCFA (the US Health Care Financing Administration, renamed in 2001 the Centers for Medicare and Medicaid Services, or CMS) modified its regulations regarding medication use by nursing home residents who are 65 years of age or older. As part of their review, surveyors will determine if the resident is taking any medications considered to have a high potential ("high severity") for severe adverse drug reactions (ADRs) or medications with a high potential for less severe ("low severity") ADRs. Residents receiving any medications will be monitored for ADRs. If an ADR is identified, the rationale for the medication use must be justified and considered appropriate. If it is not, a deficiency will be cited.

Persons wishing additional information are advised to contact the American Society of Consultant Pharmacists (see p 203 for telephone number, Web site).

The medications specified in **Table 88** are considered "high severity" by CMS and should be considered potentially inappropriate for use in treating elderly persons.

Table 88. Drugs Considered "High Severity" by CMS	
Class or Drug	**Comments**
Amitriptyline (*Elavil*)	May be used for neurogenic pain if an evaluation of risk vs. benefit of the drug is documented, including consideration of alternative therapies
Chlorpropamide (*Diabinese*)	
Digoxin, in dosages > 0.125 mg/d	Unless an atrial arrhythmia is being treated; high severity is considered if started within the past month
Disopyramide (*Norpace*)	
GI antispasmodics (belladonna alkaloids, clidinium, dicyclomine, hyoscyamine, propantheline)	Use for short periods (not over 7 d) on an intermittent basis (not more frequently than q 3 mo) does not require review by the surveyor
Meperidine, oral	If started within past month
Methyldopa	If started within past month
Pentazocine	
Ticlopidine	Review by the surveyor is not necessary in individuals who receive it because they have had a previous stroke or have evidence of stroke precursors (ie, TIAs) and cannot tolerate aspirin

The drug-diagnosis combinations specified in **Table 89** are considered "high severity" by CMS and should be considered potentially inappropriate for use in treating elderly persons.

Table 89. Diagnosis-Drug Combinations Considered "High Severity" by CMS		
Class or Drug	**Diagnosis**	**Comments**
Sedatives, hypnotics	COPD	Short-acting benzodiazepines are acceptable
NSAIDs	Active or recurrent gastritis, peptic ulcer disease, GERD	COX-2 inhibitors are not included on the list of NSAIDs
Metoclopramide	Seizures or epilepsy	
ASA, NSAIDs, dipyridamole, ticlopidine	Anticoagulation	
Anticholinergic drugs	BPH	
TCAs	Arrhythmias	If started within past month

The medications listed in **Table 90** are considered "low severity" by CMS and should be considered as potentially inappropriate in treating elderly patients.

Table 90. Drugs Considered "Low Severity" by CMS	
Class or Drug	**Comments**
Antihistamines	That is, with anticholinergic properties
Cyclandelate	
Digoxin, in dosages > 0.125 mg/d	Unless an atrial arrhythmia is being treated; high severity is considered if started within the past month
Diphenhydramine	Review by a surveyor is not necessary if used for a short time (not over 7 d) on an intermittent basis (not more frequently than q 3 mo) for allergies
Dipyridamole	
Ergot mesylates (eg, *Hydergine*)	
Indomethacin	Short-term use (eg, 1 wk) is considered acceptable for treatment of gouty arthritis
Meperidine, oral	If therapy longer than 1 mo
Muscle relaxants (eg, carisoprodol, chlorzoxazone, cyclobonzaprine, dantrolene, metaxalone, methocarbamol, orphenadrine)	Use for short periods (not over 7 d) on an intermittent basis (not more frequently than q 3 mo) does not require review

The drug-diagnosis combinations specified in **Table 91** are considered "low severity" by the CMS and should be considered potentially inappropriate in all elderly patients.

Table 91. Diagnosis-Drug Combinations Considered "Low Severity" by CMS		
Class or Drug	**Diagnosis**	**Comments**
Corticosteroids	Diabetes mellitus	If started within past month
Potassium supplements or ASA (>325 mg/d)	Active or recurrent gastritis, peptic ulcer disease, or GERD	Use of potassium supplements to treat low potassium levels until they return to the normal range is permissible if prescriber determines that use of fresh fruits and vegetables or other dietary supplementation is not adequate or possible
Antipsychotics	Seizures or epilepsy	Treatment of acute psychosis for 72 h or less is permissible
Narcotic drugs, including propoxyphene	BPH	Review by the surveyor is not necessary if use is for short duration (7 d or less) on an intermittent basis (once q 3 mo) for symptoms of an acute, self-limiting condition
Bladder relaxants (flavoxate, oxybutynin, bethanechol)	BPH	Review by the surveyor is not necessary if use is for short duration (7 d or less) on an intermittent basis (once q 3 mo) for symptoms of an acute, self-limiting condition
Anticholinergic antihistamines, GI antispasmodics, anticholinergic antidepressants, and narcotic drugs (including propoxyphene)	Constipation	Constipation can be worsened Review by the surveyor is not necessary if use is for short duration (7 d or less) on an intermittent basis (once q 3 mo) for symptoms of an acute self-limiting condition
Antiparkinson medications	Constipation	Constipation can be worsened
Decongestants, theophylline, methylphenidate, SSRI antidepressants and desipramine, MAOIs, β-agonists	Insomnia	Insomnia can be worsened

IMPORTANT TELEPHONE NUMBERS AND WEB SITES

General Information on Aging

AGS Foundation for Health in Aging	www.healthinaging.org	212-755-6810
Administration on Aging	www.aoa.gov/naic	202-619-0724
American Association of Retired Persons	www.aarp.org	800-424-3410
American Geriatrics Society	www.americangeriatrics.org	800-247-4779
American Medical Directors Association	www.amda.com	800-876-2632
American Society of Consultant Pharmacists	www.ascp.com	800-355-2727
Assisted Living Federation of America	www.alfa.org	703-691-8100
Children of Aging Parents	www.caps4caregivers.org	800-227-7294
CDC National Prevention Information Network	www.cdcnpin.org	800-458-5231
Family Caregiver Alliance	www.caregiver.org	800-445-8106
Medicare Hotline	www.medicare.gov	800-MEDICARE (800-633-4227)
National Adult Day Services Association	www.nadsa.org	866-890-7357
National Council on the Aging	www.ncoa.org	202-479-1200
National Institute on Aging	www.nia.nih.gov	800-222-2225

Elder Mistreatment

National Center on Elder Abuse	www.elderabusecenter.org	202-898-2586

End-of-Life

Last Acts	www.lastacts.org	202-296-8071
National Hospice and Palliative Care Organization	www.nhpco.org	800-658-8898 for hospice referral

Smoking Cessation

American Cancer Society	www.cancer.org (search on "quit smoking")	800-ACS-2345 (800-227-2345)
American Lung Association	www.lungusa.org	800-LUNG-USA (800-586-4872)
CDC National Center for Chronic Disease Prevention and Health Promotion	www.cdc.gov/tobacco/how2quit.htm	800-311-3435
National Cancer Institute	www.smokefree.gov	877-44U-QUIT (877-448-7848) TTY: 800-332-8615

Specific Health Problems

Alzheimer's Association	www.alz.org	800-272-3900
American Cancer Society	www.cancer.org	800-ACS-2345 (800-227-2345)
Alzheimer's Disease Education and Referral Center	www.alzheimers.org	800-438-4380
American Academy of Ophthalmology	www.aao.org	800-222-3937
American Association for Geriatric Psychiatry	www.aagponline.org	301-654-7850
American College of Obstetricians and Gynecologists	www.acog.com	800-673-8444
American Diabetes Association	www.diabetes.org	800-DIABETES (800-342-2383)

American Foundation for the Blind	www.afb.org	800-AFB-LINE (800-232-5463)
American Heart Association	www.americanheart.org	800-AHA-USA1 (800-242-8721)
American Lung Association	www.lungusa.org	800-LUNG-USA (800-586-4872)
American Obesity Association	www.obesity.org	202-776-7711
American Pain Society	www.ampainsoc.org	847-375-4715
American Parkinson Disease Association	www.apdaparkinson.com	800-223-2732
American Urological Association	www.auanet.org	410-727-1100
Arthritis Foundation	www.arthritis.org	800-283-7800
Better Hearing Institute	www.betterhearing.org	800-EARWELL (800-327-9355)
Lighthouse International	www.lighthouse.org	800-829-0500
Meals On Wheels Association of America	www.mowaa.org	703-548-5558
National Association for Continence	www.nafc.org	800-BLADDER (800-252-3337)
National Diabetes Information Clearinghouse	www.diabetes.niddk.nih.gov	800-860-8747
National Digestive Disease Information Clearinghouse	www.digestive.niddk.nih.gov	800-891-5389
National Eye Institute	www.nei.nih.gov	301-496-5248
National Heart, Lung and Blood Institute	www.nhlbi.nih.gov	301-592-8573
National Institute of Arthritis and Musculoskeletal and Skin Diseases	www.niams.nih.gov	877-22-NIAMS (877-226-4267)
National Institute of Mental Health	www.nimh.nih.gov	866-615-NIMH (866-615-6464)
National Institute of Neurological Disorders and Stroke	www.ninds.nih.gov	800-352-9424
National Institute on Deafness and Other Communication Disorders	www.nidcd.nih.gov	800-241-1044 TTY: 800-241-1055
National Kidney and Urologic Diseases Information Clearinghouse	www.kidney.niddk.nih.gov	800-891-5390
National Osteoporosis Foundation	www.nof.org	800-223-9994
National Parkinson Foundation	www.parkinson.org	800-327-4545
Self Help for Hard of Hearing People	www.hearingloss.org	301-657-2248 TTY: 301-657-2249
Sexuality Information and Education Council of the US	www.siecus.org	212-819-9770
The Simon Foundation for Continence	www.simonfoundation.org	800-23-SIMON (800-237-4666)

Page references followed by *t* and *f* indicate tables and figures, respectively. Trade names are in *italics*.

Page references followed by *t* and *f* indicate tables and figures, respectively.
Trade names are in *italics*.

Page references followed by *t* and *f* indicate tables and figures, respectively.
Trade names are in *italics*.

Page references followed by *t* and *f* indicate tables and figures, respectively.
Trade names are in *italics*.

Page references followed by *t* and *f* indicate tables and figures, respectively.
Trade names are in *italics*.

Page references followed by *t* and *f* indicate tables and figures, respectively.
Trade names are in *italics*.

Page references followed by *t* and *f* indicate tables and figures, respectively.
Trade names are in *italics*.

Page references followed by *t* and *f* indicate tables and figures, respectively. Trade names are in *italics*.

Page references followed by *t* and *f* indicate tables and figures, respectively. Trade names are in *italics*.

Page references followed by *t* and *f* indicate tables and figures, respectively.
Trade names are in *italics*.

Page references followed by *t* and *f* indicate tables and figures, respectively.
Trade names are in *italics*.

Page references followed by *t* and *f* indicate tables and figures, respectively.
Trade names are in *italics*.

Page references followed by *t* and *f* indicate tables and figures, respectively.
Trade names are in *italics*.

Page references followed by *t* and *f* indicate tables and figures, respectively.
Trade names are in *italics*.

Page references followed by *t* and *f* indicate tables and figures, respectively. Trade names are in *italics*.

Page references followed by *t* and *f* indicate tables and figures, respectively.
Trade names are in *italics*.

Page references followed by *t* and *f* indicate tables and figures, respectively.
Trade names are in *italics*.

Page references followed by *t* and *f* indicate tables and figures, respectively.
Trade names are in *italics*.

Page references followed by *t* and *f* indicate tables and figures, respectively.
Trade names are in *italics*.

Page references followed by *t* and *f* indicate tables and figures, respectively.
Trade names are in *italics*.

Page references followed by *t* and *f* indicate tables and figures, respectively.
Trade names are in *italics*.

Page references followed by *t* and *f* indicate tables and figures, respectively.
Trade names are in *italics*.

Page references followed by *t* and *f* indicate tables and figures, respectively. Trade names are in *italics*.

Page references followed by *t* and *f* indicate tables and figures, respectively. Trade names are in *italics*.

Page references followed by *t* and *f* indicate tables and figures, respectively. Trade names are in *italics*.

Page references followed by *t* and *f* indicate tables and figures, respectively.
Trade names are in *italics*.

ABOUT THE AMERICAN GERIATRICS SOCIETY

Founded in 1942, the American Geriatrics Society (AGS) is the leading clinical society devoted to the care of older adults. The AGS promotes high quality, comprehensive, and accessible care for America's older population, including those who are chronically ill and disabled. The organization provides leadership to health care professionals, policy makers, and the public by developing, implementing, and advocating programs in patient care, research, professional and public education, and public policy.

Its 6200 members include primary care physicians, geriatricians, geropsychiatrists, nurse practitioners, social workers, physician assistants, physical therapists, pharmacists, and others from the United States and around the world who are dedicated to improving the health, independence, and quality of life of the older population.

The AGS has long championed efforts to expand the national work force of clinicians with the specialized knowledge and skills to care for our aging population. Since the early 1990s, with funding from the John A. Hartford Foundation of New York City, the AGS has worked effectively to increase geriatrics expertise among subspecialists in internal medicine, practicing primary care physicians, and nonprimary-care specialists.

In 1999, the AGS reached beyond its traditional role as a professional medical society and launched the **Foundation for Health in Aging (FHA)**. The FHA aims to build a bridge between the research/practice of geriatrics health care professionals and the public, and to advocate on behalf of older adults regarding issues of wellness and preventive care, self-responsibility and independence, and connections to family and community. For more information about FHA initiatives and its' public education resources, please visit the Foundation Web site at www.healthinaging.org.

Current Major Publications and Programs of the AGS Include:

Journal of the American Geriatrics Society—rated in the top three of the ISI Science Citation Index for geriatrics and gerontology publications.

Annals of Long-Term Care: Clinical Care and Aging—This journal presents the highest quality clinical reviews, analysis, and opinions that impact the present and future of long-term care, and is the premier source of information for professionals in the long-term care market.

Clinical Geriatrics—This journal focuses on both the clinical and practical issues related to the treatment and management of older persons.

Geriatrics Review Syllabus: A Core Curriculum in Geriatric Medicine—the ground-breaking self-assessment, continuing education program for primary care providers and a premier source of clinically relevant information in geriatric medicine, now in its 5th edition.

Geriatrics Nursing Review Syllabus—the core curriculum in advanced practice geriatric nursing (GNRS), is a concise, up-to-date, and comprehensive text developed by the AGS in collaboration with the John A. Hartford Foundation Institute of Geriatric Nursing at New York University.

Geriatrics At Your Fingertips™—a comprehensive pocket-sized reference to clinical geriatrics that provides up-to-date, practical information on the evaluation and management of diseases and disorders most common to elderly people. Updated annually. Visit the Fingertips web site at www.geriatricsatyourfingertips.org.

Geriatrics Review Syllabus for Specialists—Derived from both *Geriatrics At Your Fingertips* and the *Geriatrics Review Syllabus,* this textbook focuses on the surgical approach to the elderly patient.

Public Education Publications from the Foundation for Health in Aging—FHA publishes a variety of pamphlets and tools promoting disease prevention and healthy living, as well as describing the latest knowledge about age-associated chronic illness. ***Eldercare at Home*** is an extensive guide for families involved in providing care for older relatives who want to remain at home. Information on these and other public education programs is available on the Foundation Web site.

AGS Newsletter and AGS Web site (www.americangeriatrics.org)—excellent sources of information on AGS activities and programs, noteworthy news, public policy issues, career opportunities in geriatrics, and much more.

Policy Position Statements and Clinical Practice Guidelines—In its Clinical Practice Guidelines series, the AGS has recently released a new guideline "Improving the Care of the Older Person with Diabetes Mellitus" as a supplement to the May 2003 issue of the *Journal of the American Geriatrics Society.* The AGS publishes position statements, papers, and guidelines to bring important issues in geriatrics education, research, clinical practice, and public policy to the attention of those working in the field, including policy makers, legislators, people in the health care industry, clinicians, and others.

The AGS Annual Scientific Meeting—the premier forum for the latest information on clinical geriatrics, research on aging and health, problems of older adults, and innovative models in health care delivery as well as teaching in geriatrics.

The Geriatrics Recognition Award—awarded to recognize physicians and nurses who are committed to advancing their geriatrics knowledge in order to provide better care to older adults.

The AGS Awards Program—includes the following: the Edward Henderson Award and State-of-the-Art Lecture; AGS Clinician of the Year; AGS/Merck New Investigator Awards; Pfizer/AGS Postdoctoral Fellowship Awards; Dennis W. Jahnigen Memorial Award; the Nascher/Manning Award; the Outstanding Scientific Clinical Investigator Award; the Edward Henderson Student Award; and the AGS Student Research Award.

Special Projects in Professional Education/Outreach are funded by foundations and industry sponsors.

If you would like further information about the AGS, please contact us at:

The American Geriatrics Society
Empire State Building
350 5th Avenue, Suite 801
New York, NY 10118
www.americangeriatrics.org

Call the AGS toll free at
(800) 247-4779

Send an e-mail to:
info.amger@americangeriatrics.org

GERIATRICS *At Your* FINGERTIPS
2004, 6th Edition
(ISBN 1-4051-0443-0)
From the American Geriatrics Society

A guide to the evaluation and management of the diseases and disorders that most commonly affect older persons.

Portable, Practical, Fully Indexed, and Up-to-Date!

Send completed order form with payment to:

Blackwell Publishing
c/o AIDC
PO Box 20
Williston, VT 05495-0020

For fast service
Call: 800-216-2522
Fax: 800-864-7626
Order online at www.blackwellpublishing.com/1405104430

Please send me _____ copies of *Geriatrics At Your Fingertips*, 2004, 6th Edition
@ $12.95 each

Subtotal   _____

Sales Tax (MA, VT, CA, NY and Canada)   _____

Shipping & Handling   _____
(North America: $2.50 + $1.00 ea additional
Overseas: $8.00 + $1.00 ea additional)

TOTAL   _____

To order quantities of 25 or greater please contact our special sales department at 800-759-6102 x8341.

Method of Payment: _____ Check or money order payable to Blackwell

_____ MasterCard   _____ VISA   _____ AMEX

Card Number _____ Exp.Date _____

Signature _____

Shipping Instructions (must be complete)

Name: _____
Address: _____
City: _____State: _____ Zip: _____
Phone: _____
E-mail Address: _____

Your request places you on the Blackwell e-alert electronic mailing list. You will be among the first in your discipline to find out about new releases, special offers, and textbook announcements from Blackwell. After you receive your first e-alert, you have the option of canceling the service at any time. Prices subject to change without notice.

GAYF04